## What O<sup>...</sup>

"Cindy Brynteson has a gift for taking [...] ght control and making them understandable. Her book, *You Can Live Like This* is medically sound, immensely actionable, and a foundation for sustainable, healthy living. Her balanced approach (what I call her Goldilocks style of not too much, not too little, but just the right amount of guidance) makes for a successful road map for both wellness and healthy longevity. In today's information overload world, Brynteson has distilled the advice of reputable experts and added her own life experience and that of others to serve up a feast of practical knowledge that everyone can use. This book can help you live a healthier life. The TEID Lifestyle is real, and you absolutely can live like that!"

**- J. Fon Eaker, MD, FACOG, DABOM**
Author of *Healthy Habits for a Fit Family* and *A Woman's Guide to Hormone Health*

"Having known Cindy and her husband, Jens, for quite some time, I know of their passion for their own health and for that of others. I can safely say this book is not written to make money or to become the next fad-diet craze. For those fortunate enough to read this book, Cindy shares her many years of experience and education in finding what works best for these wonderful bodies our Creator has given us. I have observed Cindy and Jens faithfully living the lifestyle she describes, and I can assure you that they are two of the healthiest people I know.

I found this book to be a delightfully easy read. It is informative and insightful. It became abundantly clear in reading the information presented in this book that this is a lifestyle our bodies were created to live by for optimum health. The facts presented in this book are backed by science. You will be blessed by the information you are about to read in this wonderful book. I suggest you read each testimonial presented here. They will inspire you to action knowing if others can do this, so can you!"

**- James Cotton, Pastor**
Spirit Alive Church

"Cindy's book, *You Can Live Like This,* will change your thinking about diets and help you realize it is completely backward! I personally know Sandi, Cindy's sister whom she talks about in her book. I have seen the transformation the TEID Lifestyle has made in her life. This book beautifully simplifies this lifestyle for you! You don't have to know the science of nutrition before beginning. She debunks the myths about diets and educates you about a healthy lifestyle.

I love her helpful guidelines and tips that you can use even when dining out to know proper portion sizes without having to smuggle food scales or measuring cups and spoons into the restaurant. Unlike so many diet fads that come and go, Cindy offers a lifestyle that is fun with creative ways to accomplish your goals! She knows that you can do this for a lifetime."

**- Robin Cannon, Head of School/Founder**
Christ Classical Academy

"If you're serious about restoring a maximal healthy balance in your lifestyle, Cindy Brynteson is the coach and living example you have been looking for. I have known Cindy and her family for over forty years. Her synthesis of sound nutritional knowledge and personal encouragement into practical balanced healthy living is what you hold in your hands. She lives it. She believes it! And she is authentically passionate for you to discover the path she is on to a more abundant life!

**- Paul Hughes, President**
Kingdom Forerunners, Inc.

"When Cindy asked me for an endorsement, I didn't think I had time. But as I read the manuscript, it became clear that this was a divine setup! As I read this manuscript, I have found the next level of health that I need to work on to live out the rest of my life.

Cindy has given us knowledge and a blueprint to help us live a healthy lifestyle and find the nutrition through the right foods and eliminate the wrong foods to live a healthy and prosperous life. I genuinely recommend this book. I believe if you invest the time to read this book, you also will walk away and say in your heart, 'this was a divine setup.'"

**- Charles L. Coker Jr. Senior Leader**
Identity Church, Deltona, Florida

"Cindy and her husband, Jens, live the principles and disciplines provided to you in an easy, demystified, step-by-step process that anyone can follow. Their passion and providence are seen throughout the fabric of their lives and this book. Most importantly, Cindy reveals the pathway to a healthy life."

**- Brian Koslow**
National Best-Selling Author

# YOU CAN LIVE LIKE THIS

## CINDY BRYNTESON, RN

*Blessings,
Cindy*

*You Can Live Like This: Teid Lifestyle*™
Copyright © 2022 by Cindy Brynteson

No part of this book may be reproduced without written permission from the publisher or copyright holder, nor may any part of this book be transmitted in any form or by any means electronic, mechanical, photocopying, recording, or other, without prior written permission from the publisher or copyright holder.

ISBNs: 979-8-9864086-0-6 (Print)

979-8-9864086-1-3 (E-book)

Printed in the United States of America.

I dedicate this book to my husband and my family:
Jens
Brad, Kara, Oliver, Everly, Arlyn, and Zoey
Danny, Nancy, Campbell, Piper, and Merlin
You make my heart full!
With all of my love,
Cindy, aka "CiCi"

# Acknowledgments

This writing has been born throughout a two-year journey. Initially, my youngest son, Danny, was my assistant. Much of the research and data collection to make my points was to his credit. Additionally, he created my tables used to break down the phases of the TEID Lifestyle. My oldest son, Brad, and his wife, Kara, were involved as I was deciphering my path with their guiding assistance. During the final writings, my sister, Sandi, whom you will read about her amazing testimony, was a great help to keep me focused and moving through the busyness of my days. She gave me some of the best critical evaluation and praise I could have asked for. Sandi walked in my shadow as my journey was beginning and later blessed me by helping to recall the precise steps we had taken.

My grandchildren, Campbell, Oliver, Piper, Everly, and Arlyn, have given me the most beautiful reasons to live a long and healthy life. It's a dream come true to be able to run and play and keep up with them. Being a part of their lives is my greatest pleasure and has brought the most incredible fun times into our lives. Every year as I watch them grow, I get even more excited about the relationship we share. Doing life together has given me the privilege to walk out my legacy with my grandchildren. Seeing life from their eyes adds much delight to my heart. I am so grateful to my children and their spouses for sharing their treasures with us.

I have been blessed to coach several through this lifestyle. My experience has confirmed the ever-increasing need for a simple plan where others can accomplish their desired weight too. Most do not begin their journey seeking healthy balance; their only goal is to lose weight. It becomes their delight to discover healthy balance is an added benefit of the TEID Lifestyle. I am forever grateful for each beautiful testimony shared within this book. It is an understatement to say my heart is full seeing how their lives have been blessed.

The prayers of faithful family and friends have given me the wisdom and strength to stay balanced and focused. This has been especially powerful on days that were packed full to the brim when I had words flowing out of me that needed to find their proper place in this book. I am so grateful for all God has shown and given me during this time, including the people He has brought into my life to accomplish this writing.

Lastly, but most importantly, my husband, Jens, has been my greatest cheerleader through it all. As we celebrate forty-six years of marriage this year, I still feel beyond blessed. I could not have accomplished this undertaking without him. His encouragement to follow the calling God has given me has driven me to look deep inside of myself. This exercise has truly brought me to know who I am, whose I am, and what I have been gifted and blessed to share with all who are looking and ready to learn. Jens is just one more example of how our family is so complementary to each other. We don't all carry the same strengths and gifts. We carry our own strengths and God-given gifts, which allow us to do great things individually and together.

# Disclaimer

*All information, recommendations, and data presented in this book reflect the individual beliefs and experiences of the author or the people being quoted. All content, including text, graphics, images, and information contained on or available through this writing is for general information purposes only. The contents of this writing are not intended as or should not be construed as "medical advice." Nor is ANY part of this book meant as a substitute for professional medical advice.*

*My position as the author of this book is that you should ALWAYS make ALL health care decisions under the direct guidance of a legitimate, knowledgeable, and experienced health care practitioner that you trust, and never just because you read something. Even the use of a nutrient supplement should be done under the direct supervision of a licensed medical practitioner. The author of this book disclaims responsibility or liability for any loss or hardship that may be incurred as a result of the use or application of any information included in this book. Information printed in this book is from sources believed to be reliable, but no guarantee, express or implied, can be made regarding the accuracy of the same. Such information is subject to change without notice. The contents of this book have not been evaluated by the Food and Drug Administration. Nothing reported or written in this book is intended to advise, diagnose, treat, cure, or prevent any disease.*

# Contents

| | |
|---|---|
| **Foreword** | **15** |
| **Preface** | **17** |
| **Chapter 1   My Story** | **21** |
| The Unexpected Gift | 21 |
| Food and Family | 22 |
| The Good Old Days | 23 |
| Unknown Pain | 26 |
| My Story Continues | 29 |
| **Chapter 2   Live At Your Optimal Weight** | **35** |
| Wake Up Your Metabolism | 35 |
| Lose Weight and Keep it Off! | 36 |
| A Word about the Science of it All | 36 |
| **Chapter 3   Sandi's Testimony** | **39** |
| **Chapter 4   Stop Blaming Yourself** | **43** |
| It's Not Your Fault | 43 |
| Why Diets Don't Work | 44 |
| A Key Reason You Can't Lose Weight | 46 |
| **Chapter 5   First Steps** | **53** |
| Make Yourself a Priority | 53 |
| Take Ownership | 55 |
| Variety Is Key | 55 |
| No More Counting Calories | 57 |
| Protein, Fat, and Carbohydrates | 57 |
| Listen to Your Body | 59 |
| The Scale Is Your Friend | 60 |
| **Chapter 6   Balance** | **63** |
| What Healthy Balance Looks Like | 63 |
| A Healthy Balance Can Produce Healing | 72 |
| Balance Means Eating Regularly | 72 |
| What about Supplements? | 73 |

## Chapter 7   Inflammation                           75

    What This Means to Your Body, and How Fat Helps     76
    Fat Defined     76
    The Digestive System     83
    Gluten     84
    Food Allergies, Sensitivities, and Intolerances     85
    Leaky Gut     86
    Autoimmune Disorders     87
    Gut Dysbiosis     88

## Chapter 8   TEID Lifestyle     91

    Planning and Prepping Defines Your Win     93
    Steps of Preparation     94
    Phase 1: TEID Lifestyle     96
    Protein Shake, a Great Way to Begin Your Day     98
    When to Begin Phase 2 of the TEID Lifestyle     100
    Phase 2: TEID Lifestyle     102
    Phase 3: the Final Phase of the TEID Lifestyle     108

## Chapter 9   Nutritional Balance Defined     111

    Organic versus Non-Organic     111
    GMO versus Non-GMO     112
    Meat     113
    Vegetables, Fiber, and Fruit     117
    Blood Sugar Balance     126
    Eating Seasonally     126
    Cleaning Produce Matters     127
    Citric Acid: it's Not What You Think it Is     128
    Herbs and Spices     130
    Sugars and Sugar Substitutes     131
    The Nutrition Facts Label     134

## Chapter 10   Nutrition Begins at Home     137

    Meal Planning and Shopping Simplified     137
    Ways to Include Your Family     140
    Phase I: Sample Menu for Seven Days     141
    Micro-Greens You Can Grow at Home     145

## Chapter 11   If These Can Do it, So Can You!     151

    Gina Merritt     151
    Katia Oliveira     152

|    |     |
|----|-----|
| Steve Merritt | 153 |
| Mia Whitt | 154 |
| Raimi Rutledge | 155 |
| Mindy Miller | 156 |
| Don Mahrer | 156 |

**Chapter 12  Stem Cells** — **157**

**Conclusion: Until We Meet Again** — **159**

# FOREWORD

We grew up in South Africa, and my (Adonica's) family generally ate in the way Cindy describes here in her wonderful book. An influential nutritionist greatly influenced my mother so, thankfully, we were never misled by the low-fat diet myth but continued to eat healthy fats and proteins, along with a great variety of fruits and raw or lightly steamed vegetables. Fruit was our dessert and our snack.

My mother made sure we had protein for breakfast and every evening for dinner. Even after a long day at her daycare center, she made dinner for us, consisting of grilled meat and two or three varieties of steamed veggies. We were privileged to live in an era when most foods were produced, grown, and raised in a much healthier manner, and none of us ever battled with our weight.

Unfortunately, when we immigrated to America, we felt like we began to lose control of our weight and our health. Because we traveled so much, we were forced to eat out much more than we would've liked to.

We realized that the food here was not as healthy as back home, but we didn't know how bad it was. The fruit in America was so much larger than the fruit in South Africa, but was paler in color and not as flavorful. We noticed that Americans generally did not eat very many vegetables, and when they did eat them they were not prepared correctly. Also, pizza and chicken nuggets seemed to be the staple foods.

Together with a faulty food pyramid, Americans were subjected to more and more genetically modified and man-made foods with countless chemical additives. Many of these additives are deliberately added to the food to cause people to become addicted to it and to purchase more of it. Because soils have been depleted of nutritional value, the nutrients in American produce is much lower than it should be.

This has resulted in a generation of people who eat way too much and yet are severely nutritionally deficient. When food is clean, organic, and grown in healthy soil, the nutrition content is higher, and we can feel satisfied with less. There is less need or temptation to eat more.

## You Can Live Like This

Today in America, we each have to take responsibility for our own health. It is not always an easy thing to do, but we must go out of our way to make sure to make good choices. They are available if we know what they are and where to find them.

You may have to forget everything you know or have been taught about nutrition and what is healthy and what is unhealthy. Cindy's book will not take long to read, but it is full of wonderful advice and sound science to help you make better choices and live a healthier, happier life!

We highly recommend this book to anyone interested in living a longer and healthier life.

**- Pastors Rodney & Adonica Howard-Browne**
Revival Ministries International

# PREFACE

Do you believe that you can live at your optimum weight, feel good, have energy, and a healthy balanced lifestyle all at the same time? If you are not 100% sure, then you are the one I have written this book for. My belief is that the TEID Lifestyle will give you the knowledge and power to accomplish your weight goals and so much more. Yes, it's a lifestyle. And building a foundation of understanding will enable you to make these lasting changes.

This lifestyle can set you free from past failures and guide you into a happier more beautiful you. None of those past failures has been wasted! Everything—yes, everything—has led you here to your discovery of health, balance, and living at your optimum weight.

Who has not asked themselves at least one of these questions?

- Why can't I lose weight?
- How do I accomplish my perfect weight?
- How can I get my metabolism to work for me, not against me?
- How do I keep the weight I have lost off, without starving myself?
- Can some foods cause me to feel pain?
- How do I live a life where food isn't in charge of me?
- What does a healthy, balanced life look like?

Do you want to know the answers? These are obtainable goals and my book is packed with a step by step guide to accomplish them. You will experience the natural progression to health and balance and find yourself living at your optimum weight.

The distractions and challenges we face daily cause us to forfeit our goals and our victory. While we have the desire, everything else has our attention, energy, and focus. Becoming the person we desire to be is constantly placed on hold, unintentionally. Many of us stay this course until life hits us. I'm sure you know all too well what I mean. We get that wake-up call from the doctor; our blood work has gone from good to bad, our blood pressure is not in a good range, or we receive a life-threatening diagnosis. For some, we just reached a point where we have become sick and tired of ourselves. We are so over the roller-coaster lifestyle of dieting and diet fads, that we are too exhausted to try just one more time. And then there are those that don't know how much more pain they can handle. The bottom line is that we hit a place of desperation. This desperation can be a good starting place. It means you are finally willing to do what it takes to live at your perfect weight, combined with a metabolism that works for you, not against you. And to begin your journey to become free of pain. I am not talking about medications, shots, or weight loss surgery. The natural way is found in the TEID Lifestyle.

When we read testimonies of others who have succeeded, we are no longer willing to allow the lies in our head to tell us that this is unobtainable for us. We no longer want to just watch everyone else live life. We want a chance to live out our lives fully and freely too. We are ready to begin our day feeling good, happy with ourselves, and excited about life.

Maybe something or someone has come into your life, giving you a reason to take your health and life seriously, and now you desire to take steps to do something about it. You are not alone. Each of us is on our best journey with different reasons to take charge of our life. If you haven't reached this place yet, then put this book somewhere in your back pocket so you can pull it out when that day comes. Most likely, there is one thing we all have in common, a desire for a change for the better. In other words, you want to feel good and be the best you that you can be, but you just haven't figured out how to do this yet.

My goal is to simplify the plethora of information out there and put the science into a simple picture with a few basic steps. These steps will show you how you can:

- Say no to yo-yo dieting
- Reach your optimum weight
- Understand how to maintain it for life
- Learn what it takes to power up your metabolism
- Live a balanced, healthy lifestyle
- Increase your energy level
- Improve your mental clarity
- Sleep better
- Eat out and choose wisely, so you still win

Whatever your age, you can choose the TEID Lifestyle! The icing on the cake is that you can experience better results in your blood work and hopefully live a long, active life. If this is not a goal, do not worry. For many of us, this is an exciting possibility. Can you imagine going to the doctor and they are baffled and ask what you are doing that has made such a difference; your blood work and/or the scale showed amazing improvement? Now that is exciting! These are normal side effects, so to speak, of the TEID Lifestyle.

What about experiencing a decrease in pain? If you experience chronic pain, this extra benefit of a healthy, balanced lifestyle will put a new kick into your step, a smile on your face, and will raise your confidence level. I know many live in pain and have learned to compensate for it or just assume there is nothing that can help. They are not aware that a simple, life-altering solution can bring relief from pain in lieu of more medication or surgeries. Some may no longer need the many medications they assumed they would be on for the rest of their life. Getting placed on new medications is common. Coming off of them is not in most instances. Of course, the decision about your need for prescribed medications will fall under the direction of your healthcare professional.

I do not take this privilege lightly that you are seeking answers and have picked up my book. Honestly, I can't wait to deliver hope, encouragement, and knowledge into your hands. I know for many of you, it has taken a lifetime to arrive here. I am glad we can finally meet. May you receive the answers and blessings you come seeking! If only I could be there beside you as you read and become excited with new, fresh hope and anticipation in your "Ah-ha moment." I can hear you saying, "What? I don't have to live like that? But I can live like this!" I pray my story and the stories of others are an answer to your prayers and that you, too, are truly blessed.

Welcome and thank you for reading along with me. I dedicate this book to you too. Let's get started on your journey!

May your joy be full, and the love you feel for yourself overflow, as you step into this new season, and blossom into the real you!

Blessings and hugs,

*Cindy*

# Chapter 1

# MY STORY

I want to take a few moments to give you a glimmer of my journey and the highlights of my life to let you see that my heart for health, nutrition, and balance is genuine. These attributes have been a part of my life for as long as I can remember. It wasn't until my adult years when I realized they were more than just characteristics of who I was but also defined my calling to give hope and encouragement to those who are looking and ready. In so many ways, these are foundational pieces I have built my health upon and now are even more important than ever as I journey through my senior years with confidence.

Someone out there needs to hear my story and how this all started with me. I know I'm not the only one who arrived somewhere they didn't expect and was amazed at what came from the unexpected. Maybe that someone is you; perhaps you can relate to my story.

## The Unexpected Gift

My story begins differently than you may expect. One year I got a kidney infection at Thanksgiving and another kidney infection at Christmas. It was *not* my favorite gift, but one I won't forget! After the holidays, I made an appointment to see my gynecologist. At that time, I didn't have a primary doctor, but I saw my gynecologist annually. In January, I felt pretty good. In February, I felt great.

Sound familiar? Once you can finally get an appointment to see your doctor, you feel amazing. All the exams looked great, and it made me feel happy! I came home thinking all was well and the two prior back-to-back kidney infections were just a fluke.

Then in March, I got another kidney infection, but this one hit me hard. I saw a local doctor, and he suggested there may be a kidney stone issue. I followed protocol for stones, but nothing changed.

What came next was a surprise. I began to feel bad. I didn't have very much appetite and would experience pain after eating. I found myself wanting to rest and sleep much more, especially during the day. This was abnormal for me as I am very active and I do not take naps during the day. I think resting and napping was my way to escape the pain and avoid how badly I was feeling.

This thought consumed my mind over the next few days: *Is there something really serious going on inside my body?*

## Food and Family

I grew up in a family that loved food, especially comfort foods that filled your belly and helped warm up your insides in the winter. I was born in Ohio, but my family moved to South Florida when I was a toddler, leaving my grandparents behind. This was very difficult for mom, dad, and me.

Our family was accustomed to one-pot meals, soups, stews, and sandwiches, likely due to coming through tough financial times when they were growing up. We always lived on a very limited budget. My mother told me that when she was growing up, there were always family members living together with them. The upstairs and basement were often full of relatives in need due to losing a spouse or other circumstances they were going through. It was common for families to take each other in without questioning if there was a room available or enough food to feed all mouths. At that time, it was less common for wives, like my grandmother and her siblings, to work outside of the home. My grandmother didn't even learn to drive until she was in her late '60s.

When my grandfather retired in the '70s, they moved to Florida. It was their dream to be near their two grown children and their growing families. I am sure that giving up shoveling snow for year-round sunshine was a great retirement gift for both of them.

I was in ninth grade when they joined us in Florida and moved into my bedroom. It was such a delight to have them with us that I don't think any of us thought twice about how I would manage sleeping on a sofa and sharing my bedroom.

Growing up as a child, I remember that my dad worked long hours. He left long before daylight, and it was normal for him to work through the day without having a lunch break, so he was famished when he arrived home.

My dad never thought our meal was complete unless it contained meat, white potatoes, maybe another vegetable, biscuits, or bread and gravy. Oh yes, and a tall glass of cold milk. Then before he fell into bed in the early evening, he would have another glass of milk and a cookie or two. On most days, dinner was his main or only meal. I liked meat, but my go-to food was a piece of fruit or a salad as I grew older.

I always wondered why my tastes and likes were a little different than the rest of my family. We are all made differently in our likes and dislikes. I loved the fresh and flavorful garden vegetables that our relatives grew in the spring and summer. The flavors especially appealed to me when they were raw.

# Chapter 1: My Story

We visited Ohio before my grandparents moved, and their neighbor had a cherry tree. I still have special memories of how fun it was to climb and pick cherries from the tree with her grandson. There's nothing quite like eating a piece of fruit that you just picked off the tree. Talk about flavor!

In today's hustle and bustle of life with more families living in the city for the convenience of commutes, I know many children have not ever picked fresh fruit off of a fruit tree or bush. Their only experience with fruit is in the produce aisle at the grocery store. I'm so thankful for my childhood experiences. They weren't the easiest of times, but I learned much about making something from nothing. I experienced true fruits and vegetables as I helped with gardening and picking from the fruit trees.

Back then, we didn't have the luxury of picking up fast food when we were running behind. Fast-food venues weren't even that common. In my early teen years, if finances allowed that week, my family would plan a Friday night outing, and we would drive twenty minutes to the new fast-food restauraunt with the big yellow arches. It was a special experience then because our budget didn't always allow for extravagant spending. I remember the doves cooing all around us, waiting for a handout. What a delight it was for my younger sisters and me to share our last bite of fries with them. Such simple fun is now a special memory.

## The Good Old Days

For those who are reading this, especially those much younger than me, it probably sounds like I lived in caveman days or was very protected as a child. You're right; it does! Times have truly changed. And to give a little more clarity, we didn't have cell phones, computers, or the Internet. We had a house phone that was a party line, meaning that you shared the line with two or three other families. Television was a luxury even though it only played black and white pictures; not a common item found in everyone's home.

I enjoyed a lot of time outside playing, running, riding a bicycle, or playing baseball. Many of our relatives followed suit after our move to Florida, so I spent most of my early childhood playing with my cousins who were all boys and lived a few houses away from us in the same neighborhood. Thus, I became a tomboy. I did have one girlfriend named Ann who lived down the road—the dirt road, that is.

One memory Ann and I probably have ingrained in our brains, other than our lifelong friendship, was when I convinced her to close her eyes while riding her bicycle. At that age, I wasn't thinking about the fact that she hadn't been playing cops and robbers on her bike with the boys as I had. Poor Ann ran into a cactus, and it wasn't a pretty sight! I feel so blessed that our friendship continued and still exists today.

I need to expound on what cops and robbers are in case you missed this fun game during your childhood. We, as the robbers, would ride our bikes and hide a rock in someone's mailbox. The cops had to find the rock, and then it was up to them to chase us down on a bicycle. Can you imagine kids playing this game today? Not only was it an acceptable neighborhood game, but the neighbors laughed along at the fun we were all having. Maybe that is what is meant by "the good old days"!

## Grammie

I spent a good part of my early childhood with my great aunt, who we lovingly called Grammie. She was my cousin's grandmother and my grandmother's older sister. Grammie and Chuckie had retired to South Florida before I was born. They introduced us to Florida. When my family decided to make a location change, it was the obvious answer. My mother had always lived near her family, so it became the best option for the three of us.

Grammie babysat me every day while my mom went to work at the telephone company as a telephone operator. I stayed with them regularly during the daytime until I entered elementary school. Grammie taught me about manners, how to eat roast beef, homemade bread, mashed potatoes, and vegetables from the garden after picking and preparing them, and how to finish a meal with ice cream and a homemade cookie. I can still picture her in the kitchen cooking away. She made this same meal almost every day. It was what her husband loved.

Since my grandparents had not yet moved to Florida, Grammie was my surrogate grandmother. She taught me many things that she was so good at. When she gardened, she taught me to put tin pans on a string hanging off of the fence post above the tomatoes so that the birds got frightened away instead of eating our tomatoes. She taught me how to let grandchildren do things that mom and dad didn't like. (You will understand soon enough, nothing dangerous, of course, just pure fun.)

My cousins and I would go to her home to make mud pies in a bucket. But there was only one thing we needed to complete the pretend cooking and stirring—a stick to stir the mud pies with. Grammie had nice yardsticks that we borrowed and broke in half to use for mixing our mud pies. This went on for quite some time until Grammie had had enough of getting new yardsticks every week. One day she hid in the bushes and came around the corner of the house to grab the yardstick out of my cousin's hand. Then she chased us around the house with the yardstick, waving it in the air. I know she wasn't happy, but it turned into good old-fashioned laughter and fun that still warms my heart as I think about it today. Boy, did she have a lot of patience! (And by the way, if she caught us, she would have only hugged us and laughed.)

Grammie taught me how to sew and make my clothing, which came in quite handy when I entered middle school and needed school clothes. Our family income was challenged to keep up with the current bills, especially since there were three of us girls by this time. Learning to sew made a big difference. Grammie also taught me how to make the best homemade bread and cookies. Everything was made from scratch in her home.

## Chapter 1: My Story

**Lessons Learned**

Grammie's husband was a retired barber, so she always cut my hair and gave me my annual hair perm to curl my hair. This was something my mother loved, but me, not so much. Because of this experience, I learned how to cut hair and do my hair perms.

After I was married, my husband went away for a day hunting trip. When he arrived home late that night, I greeted him at the door with a new hairdo. As I look back, it was really funny, but at the time, it was borderline hysteria on my part. I had decided that I hadn't curled my hair in so long that maybe it would be a great style to revisit. Long story short, the hair rods I used were extremely small, so I ended up with kinky little curls all over my head. If you pulled my hair down to my shoulders, it bounced right back into position into kinky tight curls. I guess you could say that I did a very good job. Ha!

I called my girlfriend Robin and told her what had happened. Our son, Bradley, was a toddler, and he was napping, so I asked my friend if she would come over to help me fix my hair. I was at a loss with my hair all kinked up and asked her to cut my hair into a nice rounded style. I didn't know what else to do. When my husband took one look at me, he asked, "Have you been to a hairstyling convention?" Oh, the memories and laughter we still have over that one! Robin is still my very good friend, too, and we have not stopped helping each other out with hairstyle ideas—and more. Just ask our husbands!

Speaking of hair reminded me of another story. When my husband and I started dating, I had very long hair down to my waist. Soon after, during my college days, I worked at a bank for one year as a teller. It was a fun job, and I met some lovely people. It was a wonderful way for me to learn about the banking world and earn enough money to get myself through nursing school.

One day a coworker told me that a hair salon had just opened across the street from the bank. The owner was a guy who was well-known in the styling world. She asked me if I wanted to go to the salon with her during our lunch break if she could get us both appointments at the same time. Well, of course, I did. If this guy was that good, this was something any girl would not want to miss out on. So we boogied on over to the Foxy Lady at noon. I was open to whatever suggestions this amazing hairstylist thought would make me look cuter.

The guy immediately suggested a style he thought would look great on me. He told me to hold my head forward, and he would cut my hair kind of in a V shape from my temples to the center back of my hair and bring the length up a little bit. It ended up being more like a "big bit!" He thought it would complement the shape of my face and said it was a new "in" style. I thought for a moment about how long it took my hair to dry, how much time I could save, and the fun of a new style and said, "let's do it."

Remember, this was during my lunch break, and I didn't have much time to think it through. My friend and I failed to tell the stylists that we only had our lunch hour. We arrived back at the bank about thirty minutes late, which was quite a big deal, especially to the others waiting to eat their lunch who were ravenous. Not to mention that we missed eating lunch in place of looking fabulous. Well, just as quickly as they got upset, they calmed down and admired our new hairstyles and hurried off to lunch. We did get a little scolding from our supervisor, but she was such an awesome lady that she understood the delay that can happen in a hair salon. Well, at least she acted sweet about it and told us not to ever do that again.

When my boyfriend (who is now my husband) stopped by the bank to cash his paycheck that afternoon, he saw my hair and was a *little* surprised. But probably not as surprised as when I walked down the church aisle on our wedding day (three-and-a-half years later), after cutting my hair myself the night before. It had grown down to my waist again, and I decided after our rehearsal dinner that my hair would be easier to manage during our honeymoon if I just pulled it around and snipped a few inches off. You know, just a short nine inches. I am so thankful my husband loved me for who I was and not my hair! That could have been a really bad-hair day for sure. He just smiled and glowed as I walked down the aisle, saving the haircut discussion for later. These memories serve me best as lots of laughter and crazy stories to share and, of course, the lessons I have learned.

You are probably wondering why I would share all of these silly stories. What do they have to do with this book? Well, I want you to see that I am a real person, mostly balanced, as you will read later. But at times, I need to get back in balance too. We all do. I also want you to see that humor and not taking yourself too seriously can be *very* important. Life is meant to be joyful—abundantly joyful! I can be very serious, but I try to keep laughter and joy alive. Our five grandchildren keep us in stitches all the time—and that helps maintain my healthy balance and makes me feel so much younger.

So let's skip ahead to the part of the story I wanted to share with you.

## Unknown Pain

A few years back, I was traveling between Georgia and Florida frequently. My mother was living in South Florida again. Her health had been failing, and my sisters and I were trying to relocate her to central Florida so she would be closer to everyone. We hoped she would be placed in a residence to help meet her needs, which would be better for her than living alone. It was a long process, but we finally got her moved into a senior living residence. We spent three weeks to set up her apartment, trying to make it feel like home. Unexpectedly, she passed away over the 4th of July weekend.

My sisters and I understand how difficult the season of helping someone in need or being a caregiver can be. And then when you lose a parent, there can be such a void in your life with many emotions to filter through. It can be challenging to focus, especially on your own needs, during this kind of journey.

# Chapter 1: My Story

For quite some time, I struggled with my health and pushed myself to be there for my mom. My sisters and I were all taking turns traveling to help her. It was difficult for me to make myself a priority while trying to help meet her needs.

At one point, my health got the attention of both my husband and I. Much later I learned that the pain I was compensating for was causing crazy rises in my blood pressure. Thank goodness I didn't settle for just taking medication for blood pressure! You will see the value of this point as you read on.

As I struggled with the pain, I kept looking for the root problem. Several months following my mother's death, new symptoms arose, and my pain increased. I had a kidney infection regularly, as you read in the previous chapter. If you have ever experienced this, it can become quite frustrating. I was given round after round of antibiotics—something I rarely take. As I mentioned, I decided to visit Dr. Eaker, my gynecologist in Augusta, Georgia, for a check-up. He is a friend of my husband and I, and we trust his opinion immensely. He examined me, did my normal annual checks, and we left, thinking, "Well, I guess nothing's going on or my body repaired itself."

A few weeks later I wasn't feeling well at all. The pain was located in my back and upper right side of my diaphragm area, which I assumed were my kidneys again. But this time the pain level had gone up a few notches. When I saw my doctor again, he thought it was a problem with my gallbladder.

To summarize two weeks of tests and blood work, I was diagnosed with an ovarian tumor, but Dr. Eaker didn't think it was causing my pain. As most of you know, having access to the internet makes us all more aware of the positive and negative possibilities that exist. My blood work for ovarian cancer showed only a slight risk for cancer, and my doctor didn't think it was a cancerous tumor. Knowing that ovarian cancer is a silent killer, I was anxious to know for sure. Generally speaking, ovarian cancer can reveal itself when cancer has metastasized. You seek help for the pain while not knowing ovarian cancer is the cause.

After the two weeks of testing, Dr. Eaker decided to remove the ovary and tumor and also do an exploratory of my pelvic and abdominal area because everything else was coming up with little or no answers from all the countless tests.

What I "enjoyed" (an oxymoron) was that the medical staff who ran scans or did diagnostic tests kept questioning me as to my birth date. My insides looked younger to them than my actual age, and they thought it was a misprint. In the midst of feeling like I could be dying, this little encouragement gave me a little hope that maybe what was going on was simpler than my imagination was now beginning to offer me.

## You Can Live Like This

**The Past Revisited**

The day of my surgery came quickly, thanks to my doctor and his diligence to keep things moving forward. After four or so hours of surgery, he met my husband, Jens, in the waiting room. He asked, "When was Cindy in a bad car accident?"

My husband replied that I had never been in a bad car accident, and then he remembered that I had been stampeded by people at a convention several years prior. Dr. Eaker went on to show him the pictures of how my insides were filled with scar tissue, and that was the culprit of my pain, which I later understood was the cause of my compromised kidney, high blood pressure from dealing with the pain, and the inflammation affecting my health.

When Dr. Eaker woke me following surgery, he was wearing a smile. It was a relief to hear that all was good, and he had removed only one ovary with the tumor, released the scar tissue, and had pictures to show me on my upcoming visit. As I digested that information over the next few days, I realized that it was all very, very minor in the scope of what could have been much worse. I felt beyond blessed, grateful, and happy to know these results.

After my recovery, which went well for a while, I slowed down and rested more than expected. It seemed that my body was taking longer to regain a normal energy level. I rested and pushed a little when I could. I am normally a high-energy person, so I figured that maybe age or undergoing hours of anesthesia was the culprit; ultimately, I just was not recovering as quickly as I anticipated and wanted to sleep a lot.

Then came the time to deal with other symptoms that I had preoperatively. These symptoms didn't seem to be connected to the ovarian issue. I had shooting pain in my head that would come and go regularly. So I was sent to see a neurologist following post-op recovery. They ordered a brain scan, and nothing showed abnormal.

After multiple other tests, I was diagnosed with neuropathy in all extremities, occipital neuropathy, damage to my neck and lower back, which was most likely all from the fall during my stampede incident. The neurologist planned for me to see a rheumatologist for further diagnosis of what form of autoimmune disease I might have. I was offered a handful of pain medication prescriptions, follow-up appointments, and referral appointments.

At this point, I started doing a form of stretching at home. The stretching and deep breathing helped me balance out the pain that was returning little by little. I thought, *We took care of the problem, so why is my pain returning?* I seriously didn't want to revisit that degree of pain! I had not anticipated the pain returning, instead, I expected this to be gone and the issue resolved. As a result, I was feeling a little confused about my healing process.

I told the neurologist that day that I didn't want the prescriptions he offered, and he became offended. He asked me if I planned to fix myself with yoga or exercise, and I answered that stretching, breathing, and relaxing exercises had been a go-to before surgery and I was now using them again to get relief. When feeling good, I normally love to do

# Chapter 1: My Story

stretching and exercise, especially while listening to praise music. During this season it helped me refocus my mind and get some relief and balance.

He told the nurse to give me a follow-up appointment and the prescriptions. He stated that I could get used to the fact that I would be seeing him regularly. I told him that I did not come for medications, I came to find more answers and to be sure that I didn't have another unknown issue or a brain tumor. My father died at the age of sixty with glioblastoma, a form of brain cancer. I never felt that I had brain cancer, but at the same time, I didn't know the source of the shooting pain in my head. I then proceeded to explain that I wanted to take ownership of my health and understand what I could do to help my body naturally strengthen and repair itself as much as possible.

Obviously, I needed to reduce inflammation if I had pain and possibly a so-called autoimmune disorder. I did not desire to live dependent on medication and was concerned that these prescriptions could cause me to need more medication for the side effects of the first drugs. I saw this play out in my mother's life with all of the pain and illness she suffered for many years and the constant changing of medication to try to get her relief.

It was clear that the doctor and I were not on the same page. I understand the reason for this. I was just one of the hundreds of patients who came to him hoping that medicine would give them some relief and possibly even quality of life.

Fortunately for me, I don't think that way. My mind thinks, *If something is out of balance and causing an issue, what can I do to feed or help my body to do what it was miraculously created to do—keep itself healthy and well?* So began a new season in my journey to discover what my body and other knowledgeable doctors would help me to understand. I wanted the big picture. I searched out alternative and natural treatments that were available beyond just taking a pill. I wasn't afraid to learn more or do whatever it took to be healthy and free of this growing pain.

## My Story Continues

My research turned up many opportunities. They all promised to offer me help. I had one phone consultation after another with medical and alternative healthcare professionals all over the southeast USA, and I believed I could find the answer and help I was desperately seeking. I knew that I had to work with someone who understood the body inside out and proved to know how important nutrition and balance would be for my healing—someone who offered more than a pill for pain. This person would help me find the path to help my body reduce inflammation, which I knew, in turn, would help reduce my pain and improve my overall health.

I chose a health and wellness clinic that came highly recommended by my family. They were the only practice, after *multiple* consultations over the next couple of months, who seemed to be coming from a whole-body perspective. She also used several of the treatments I had researched and thought might be good options for my healing process.

Because we were making a six-hour round trip to see her, my husband decided that he should also see her for some small ongoing physical issues he was struggling with. We began with examinations, physical history, and blood work. They offered a great balance of medical health combined with alternative health and we both found this quite enlightening. It confirmed, once again, how valuable a blend of medical and alternative medicine can be.

Much of the lab work wasn't the normal run-of-the-mill testing. They delved intentionally and specifically. We were surprised by the diagnosis that we each received. It was believed that my scar tissue had returned, and testing showed I did not have an autoimmune issue; I was dealing with long-term inflammation from the previous injury and damage to my body from my accident many years prior. My husband on the other hand was showing autoimmune symptoms, and they confirmed this with further extensive lab work.

There were several familiar things in our treatment, such as applied kinesiology, a form of chiropractic practice, natural supplementation for specific issues, and nutrition. Then there were things I had read about, cold lasers being an example. Within two weeks of our visits, we were both seeing some improvements.

After several months we realized the rest of our treatment plan was going to revolve around our nutrition and changes only we could implement. We planned to continue with less frequent checkups and change to a routine follow-up. In general, we were healthy eaters. So we were surprised to learn that there were some culprits hidden in our daily diets that were, most likely, adding to each of our inflammatory issues. Other than the obvious ones, we each had to discover what those were.

## Origin of My Love for Health and Nutrition

I knew early on in my childhood years that I wanted to be a registered nurse (RN). I was a candy striper as a teenager for three years. Even had the privilege to be voted the candy striper queen in my tenth-grade year of high school. I worked at Publix as a cashier for a year following my high school graduation, which allowed me to go to college during the day and work nights and weekends. The heavy schedule didn't throw me off because I had worked since sixth grade, babysitting every day after school and many weekends. I had been working one job or another for as long as I could remember and I did it to help out and be able to go to college.

I loved being around people and enjoyed most of my jobs, including my year of banking experience following being a cashier at Publix.

Then a year later, while still in college, I began working at a local hospital to further my medical knowledge and hands-on experience to become an RN. Working in the medical

## Chapter 1: My Story

field gave me familiarity with healthcare and confidence in myself as I grew and matured. My family nor I had been around the medical field growing up; my only connection was when my grandfather had coronary artery surgery during my senior year of high school when he experienced a stroke and never recovered. It was a very traumatic time for my mother and our family as they decided to turn off life support.

The only other experience I had with the medical industry came two years later when my father's mother had a heart attack and passed quickly after admission to intensive care. I remember going to see her when I got out of my college class that night and hearing that she had already passed. Looking back, I can see how both of these experiences added more fuel to my desire to be a nurse.

These activities helped me become acclimated to the medical atmosphere. I loved everything about the opportunity to learn and help people get well or bring them comfort. I had a wonderful nutrition teacher and several incredible nursing instructors in college who had a part in formulating my love for understanding how the body works and how nutrition and balance play a strong role in our health. They were a bit old-school, you might say.

After graduating as an RN, I worked on medical, psychiatric, surgical, and orthopedic floors, and then ended up in ICU and CCU. This was truly my favorite part of hospital work up to that point. I loved being a nurse to critically or acutely ill patients; working alongside the doctors, supporting the families of these patients as well as the daily challenges in the critical care setting. I even enjoyed dealing with death and dying and helping to bring comfort and peace to my patients, their families, or teaching and helping to make plans for rehabilitation.

My opportunities to grow and learn were never-ending. I became very good at making quick and accurate assessments. You may only have a minute to make a call of what to do in a critical-care setting. I wasn't hesitant to question the doctor about something he ordered; I saw myself as a second set of eyes when it came to combining medicines or ordering different tests, etc. The bottom line was that I wanted what was in the best interest and welfare of the patient.

Later I went to work for three surgeons who trained me and two other nurses. We were known as physician assistants before what we know today as a PA. My skills in this role continued to be strengthened, and I learned so much, not only from the doctors but also from the other PAs in our office. Over the years I have received certification for nutritional coaching too. But overall, I have always felt my education as an RN was the best foundation I could have had to understand the body, nutrition, health, and balance.

During my father's battle with brain cancer, which was a very small segment of time, my husband and I received a new appreciation for the balance of medical care combined with alternative and integrative medicine. I was reminded of how amazing the human body is and that, when fed properly, it can do many things to help itself. Our bodies are created with processes to help us fight against illness and disease. They can get out of balance and, in some instances, can cause our body to attack itself, causing further inflammation and illness. At a cellular level, inflammation is generally the first thing to happen with imbalance. We may not see cellular inflammation but we see the results of it when it becomes an illness, disease, or pain down the road. I was convinced about the power of nutrition—good or bad—and the results each brings.

**Back to My Journey**

So after receiving treatment, my husband and I were beginning to see improvement. If we were going to improve and create a healthier balance for ourselves, some things would need to happen. We were being encouraged to figure out what our bodies needed, didn't like, or maybe what our bodies were just tolerating and needed a break from.

I have never been a fast-food junkie nor had I made the majority of my family's meals from processed, packaged foods. My original complaint was pain, which we believed was connected to cellular inflammation. It was obvious we needed to make some intentional changes to reduce inflammation. This would be my first step as I took ownership of my nutrition and health.

I wasn't much of a dairy person as it didn't sit well with my stomach. I had already cleaned up our nutrition from the white stuff (white sugar and white flour) a few years before. But something was still missing. Since nutrition and getting to the root of things has always been one of my biggest passions and my husband enjoys it, too, we decided to take this on together. As we researched nutrition and the different styles of eating, my husband's diagnosis of an autoimmune disease caused us to look closely at what was already out there. We found so many references that taught in-depth about how you can help your body become stronger. We read that you can either halt the progress of autoimmune diseases or, in some cases, overcome them.

My sister Sandi just happened to call us that day as we were leaving our appointments. I shared with her that I was going to begin my journey by researching what was already available. Sandi asked me a lot of questions as my husband and I drove back home. Little did I know that she made a commitment to follow every step that we took. She walked closely beside us for the next several months. We didn't live in the same state at that time, but we found many ways to stay connected, sharing meal plans and every droplet of knowledge as we journeyed. Whatever I did, she did. We experimented and created recipes daily. We would journal everything and strive for answers.

One of the conclusions we both quickly agreed on was that, in general, most people might have difficulty beginning their journey with science and in-depth teaching. The answers come by leaving no stone unturned, and knowledge of the body is covered so thoroughly that one could feel they have earned a medical degree by the time they finish

## Chapter 1: My Story

researching! But overall, it proved invaluable for me. I learned so much, and my memory and knowledge of the body and how it functions was refreshed.

In this book, you won't find all of the fads, diets, and programs out there, even though I have studied them. We all know the list goes on and on. My point here is to help you understand for yourself how important *balance* is. This is such a key factor. I have been saying this for years, but it wasn't until I had the issues when I had to really practice what I preached.

I followed the various recommendations I found for a few months. I listened to the doctor as she encouraged me to listen to my body and act accordingly. Now I had someone with other medical knowledge saying the same thing to me that my mind and body had been telling me. It was fuel to my journey: to find answers. So I took what I learned and wrote a program that suited my husband, my sister and her husband, and myself. Little did I know that it was going to work incredibly well for the many others we would share with!

I was looking for balance, health, and wellness, and a way to reduce pain. I was not focused on weight loss, although thinking back, it would have been good for me to lose a few pounds. Knowing what I know about the body, I anticipated that my pain would decrease as a result, and our health would automatically improve. So I moved out confidently, but was not aware of the depth of where my journey would take all of us.

I began to create my own plan, which is actually a lifestyle I knew we could live with. As I took this journey, others started to ask questions and wanted to know what I was doing. Those who knew that I was on a journey to end my pain and improve my husband's health asked the most questions.

As you read the testimonies in my book, you will see many symptoms that the TEID Lifestyle has helped. It became like a wildfire growing among my family, our friends, and acquaintances. Those I had shared my new lifestyle with were becoming more active, energized, healthy, balanced, losing weight, and more youthful in energy, looks, and mindset—especially cognitive function. And best of all, *they turned past dieting failures into success and balance* after years of frustration and disappointment!

This is how the creation of the TEID Lifestyle came about. **TEID is the word *diet* spelled backward, and it is about unraveling the terrible confusion and past failures many have experienced while trying to stay the course of a diet.** It is intended to open the door to living the healthy, balanced lifestyle you dream of. I feel so blessed to have helped so many, but my greatest honor is to have helped my family. My middle sister spent her life struggling for balance in weight and trying to kick-start her metabolism. I can't wait for you to read her success story that just keeps living on and on! The title of this book came from her. She kept telling me, "I can't believe I don't have to live this way any longer!" So I am happy to tell you that **you can live like this!**

# Chapter 2

# LIVE AT YOUR OPTIMAL WEIGHT

I desire to be a carrier of truth and to help you know that you can live here. You can live at your desired and perfect weight. It is the way you were meant to live: in balance. The great news is that living at your desired weight doesn't need to be a battle you contend with daily. This lifestyle is your opportunity to live outside of the limited mindset the world has taught you to live in. Come on; let's get started on this journey to your freedom!

## Wake Up Your Metabolism

"My metabolism doesn't seem to be working. Is it possible to get it working *for* me instead of *against* me?"

*This is the million-dollar question asked today.* If you haven't heard anything else from my writing thus far, please hear this; you can resuscitate, kick-start, rev up, or boost your metabolism. You can set and reach a balanced, healthy, optimum weight for yourself. I have always said, "We didn't get this way overnight, so we are not going to fix ourselves in a day." It becomes a journey of breaking old habits and forming new ones.

But instead of focusing on your old habits, we will focus on what you are going to do, and these will automatically become your new habits. I believe that this is made simple by following the TEID Lifestyle. I want to be able to live a fun, pain-free, balanced, healthy lifestyle. For my own needs I created a plan that would allow me to **achieve or maintain my optimum weight and enjoy a healthy, balanced lifestyle at the same time!** You can choose this opportunity for yourself too.

You will learn in Chapter 5 that there are a few key implementations and suggestions to help your metabolism wake up. They are also the key ingredients to a healthy balance in your body. Then in Chapter 6, you will read further about balance and what it means in the TEID Lifestyle.

# You Can Live Like This

What person, especially a woman, does not desire to have her metabolism work for her instead of against her? Your metabolism must work efficiently to get to your desired weight and stay there. Otherwise, you are still living on the hamster wheel. We have to feed our bodies and give them what they need to get going and rev up. It is basic and simple once you understand it.

## Lose Weight and Keep it Off!

So many people are shocked to learn what our food today is composed of. The additives that we consume (for some in every meal) are detrimental to our bodily systems. They confuse our bodies and can be the cause of cellular inflammation. Cellular inflammation is better defined in Chapter 7, but for simplicity's sake in this chapter, inflammation increases the speed of aging and disrupts a healthy balance throughout our body. Disruption of this healthy balance can keep you from many goals, especially losing excess weight.

I, for one, get frustrated when a doctor or counselor says that we just have to accept something or that this is the way life will be from now on. No! I want everyone to know that *you don't have to live that way anymore!* I hope many of you will share this announcement. It's time we know the truth about how our bodies function and what we can do to help our bodies find health and balance. You can live with confidence in yourself and feel good about your choices.

As you learn these simple steps to retrain and reset your body, you will be astounded at how simple it is. You may even get a little angry over the ways we have been misled. But don't stay there long; move ahead to where you want to go!

## A Word about the Science of it All

Instead of explaining to you all the science of how good nutrition wakes up your metabolism, let me say that following the TEID Lifestyle will be the beginning of waking up your metabolism. Many of us don't know what dense nutrition (food filled with nutrients our bodies need) and good healthy nutrition are, and assume that good nutrition can be found in fast or processed foods. Then we load our plates with all of it, day after day. Advertisements are full of information to assist companies to boost their sales. In turn, we believe the ad and believe that the food must be good for us. Without the proper knowledge, we don't realize many ads are simply marketing tools and not proper teaching tools.

Over the years, so many preservatives have transferred from a food source to being created in a chemical lab. Most people are unaware that these forms of preservatives and additives are in our food. They mess with our food and bodies, confusing our systems and preventing them from functioning at their optimum potential. Many times these harmful substances even increase inflammation in our bodies.

# Chapter 2: Live At Your Optimal Weight

Let's get the basics down and come back to the science, if and when you want to learn more. Let's take one step at a time. I have purposefully kept this part basic and simple so you have an overview but won't feel like you have to be educated to move forward. Don't let anything hold you up! Get what you need and keep moving forward. Build your ladder of success. The main thing is to get to the main thing—what foods you are going to eat for the first thirty days or more and how to prepare yourself, your environment, and your mind for success.

The TEID Lifestyle is intended to give you steps to arrive at your optimal weight and a plan to create a healthy balance you can live in. It is very basic, simple, and doable. Once you arrive at your optimal weight, follow the Reintroduction and Phase 3. After this season, if you get off track or feel a need to tighten up your boundaries, you will have a simple plan to realign yourself back into balance. Living a balanced, healthy life results in arriving at and living at your optimal weight.

# Chapter 3

## SANDI'S TESTIMONY

My sister Sandi went through an amazing transformation when she began her own journey to health and wellness. Here is her story.

\* \* \*

I'm excited to share my journey with you to a *healthy life*! I am a wife, a mom, a grandma, and I am approaching my senior years. This could be a sad story, but I am thrilled to tell you that it is not. It's a proven story of real-life to let you know that you are never too old to learn and make changes, especially when turning your health and weight toward a positive direction and finding balance in life. I want to share my journey with you so you can see the difference in my life.

I remember how I turned to food for comfort at a very young age. As young as elementary school, I remember coming home from school to an empty house. My parents had to work, my older sister was not home from school yet, and my younger sister was with the babysitter. Being home alone was very scary for me, and I learned then that food was a comfort. As years passed, I still turned to food for comfort whenever life threw me a curveball. I never knew how to make good food choices as a child or a young adult, so my desire to learn healthy balance in my diet was huge when this opportunity presented itself.

Did I need to lose weight? Yes! I was obese because of the food choices I had made along my pathway in life. I had tried so many things and spent so much money in an attempt to lose weight. But in the end, I was never taught the right balance in making food choices. I had some success, but unfortunately, it was never lasting success. It actually made each journey even more complicated because of the increase of weight gain from each of my previous frustrations. I became more confused about what was a good choice with so many different teachings. My burning desire to learn good nutrition was never met. This can play havoc on your emotional state, as if we don't already have enough to deal with.

So in my senior years, I can finally say with great confidence and excitement that *I now have healthy nutrition and balance in my life!* This is where my sister Cindy's story and her journey have changed my life forever too! I can't begin to share with you the feelings of self-worth, achievement, happiness, and positivity this success has given me.

I finally found what I had searched for my entire life. By learning and implementing the TEID Lifestyle and all of the healthy balance she describes in this book, my body is working for the better—and it is working for and with me! My metabolism now works for me; not against me. I went from plus-size clothes to regular sizes. I no longer have a closet full of various sizes to choose from. Now I have one size in my closet. As I continue on this beautiful journey, I share the clothes with others in need as soon as I no longer fit in the ones that are too large.

My blood work is no longer out of balance. I am proud to say that it is very good. I still laugh at the memory of stepping onto the scale in the doctor's office just a month or so after I began this journey with my sister. The nurse asked me to step off so she could adjust the scale. I stepped off and she adjusted it and then reweighed me. She had the funniest look on her face. When the doctor came in, she said, "The nurse said the scale was broken."

I commented that it looked correct to me.

With sarcasm in her voice, she said, "Well, that would mean that you have lost forty pounds since I last saw you four months ago."

I said, "Well, that is right!"

She asked, "What are you doing?" I shared it with her. She looked at me like a deer in headlights. I looked at her and realized that she had not taken off her weight from having a baby a few years ago, and this program could help her too. So I began excitedly to share with her in more detail.

At that point, she wasn't ready to hear what I had to share; she wasn't desperate enough. It's the same way I used to be. Before that time, I wasn't desperate enough to listen and make some changes, not a quick fix. Then I finally got off of the roller coaster of dieting. My emotions and health are no longer at risk. It is amazing how many areas of my life have been affected over my lifetime from me being overweight, but no more!

Here is another key point. You can't let other people's doubts affect your own plans. That doctor's inability to accept what I knew to be beneficial for her, didn't throw me out of balance because she wasn't ready. I have had to deal with skepticism at times, but because of my success as early as the first few weeks, I chose not to be distracted. I learned how to make myself a priority. I'm in for life—*my life!*

# Chapter 3: Sandi's Testimony

My main goal for so many years was to eat healthily. I knew if I could achieve this, the weight would come off. It was a total surprise when the cravings and desire for carbohydrates and sugar disappeared too. It is wonderful to go on vacation. And yes, when I splurge a little too much (as we all do at times), I come home with a couple of extra pounds. But knowing that I have a simple, healthy plan in place to get it off and get back on track and in balance is the best feeling of all. Years ago I would have gone on vacation and gained back all the weight I had lost. Now that I have learned what a healthy balance looks like, I only come home with a few extra pounds that are off in a few days.

My sister mentioned earlier that maybe something is happening in your life to give you a new desire for health and balance. Well, let me tell you about my grandson! He wasn't the only reason for my changes, but I want to be able to run and play with him; to be free of pain and feel good about myself so I can pour everything well into him. I want him to learn healthy food choices as a toddler so that he, too, can experience a healthy life.

Are you ready for a change? Who or what is your reason to choose health and balance?

It's never too late to make the change! I have lost seventy-seven pounds and I consider myself a progress in the making. Nothing would be more exciting for us than to hear your testimony too!

**BEFORE**

**AFTER**

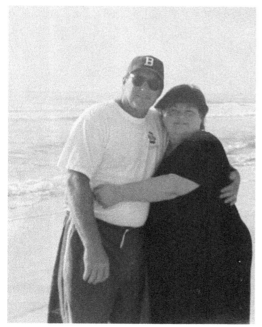
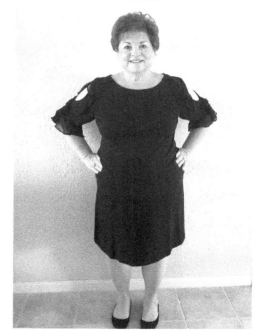

# Chapter 4

# STOP BLAMING YOURSELF

At our inner core, most of us blame ourselves for our failures. We will beat ourselves up day in and day out, even subconsciously. When we don't stop this personal abuse, indirectly, we let the constant stress and battle hinder our success. Unfortunately, our emotions take the biggest hit when we do this. Thus, the emotional roller coaster is being fueled for this ever-increasing downward journey of self-worth.

Let's agree right here and now to resolve this negative and weak way of encouraging ourselves to do better. Negativity never encourages you to go to a higher level of yourself. It also doesn't recognize or remind you that exactly what you need lies inside of you. You were created to live a healthy, balanced life. Take this *blaming* mindset and kick it out. As you place it outside the door of your mind, lock the door behind you and throw away the key. Then replace the blaming mindset with a knowledge of your high worth and high value. It might feel awkward for a bit, but this is where you are stepping into the truth of who you are and where you are supposed to live.

### It's Not Your Fault

You may have picked up this book for pleasure reading, from a recommendation, or in hopes that you will find an answer to your frustrations. Either way, I believe the chances are strong that you will find some similarities between your story and one of the testimonies I have included. I pray this confirms that there is something here for you too. I understand the need and frustrations of getting help, especially when you don't understand what caused your problem in the first place. It might be genetics, a serious illness, an accident, pain, obesity, disease, lack of mental clarity, or lack of energy, to name a few. The list could go on and on, but if you are willing to keep reading and do what it takes to help get your body on a path to balance, you will see a new you. I can't wait to hear your testimony of success too!

For many, your emotions are most likely very involved with how your body feels or how you feel about yourself. I have seen this on many occasions as I have coached others. Let me help you find peace right off the bat and get rid of any guilt or shame you may be carrying in this one simple statement: ***It's not your fault!*** Many of us have been taught the wrong information.

I want you to have a simple understanding of the basics of how your body works and responds. A scientific understanding is not quite as important right now unless that is how your brain operates. If it is simple, you can keep moving forward into a successful lifestyle without getting hung up, frustrated, and distracted with more details than you are looking for at this time. I would guess that right now you just want help and answers so that you can begin your journey too. Your belief system is most likely not trained to believe that you can and will be successful. But I am here to tell you that *you can and will do it!* If we can do it, *so can you!*

> **Correct knowledge can help you break through your limiting beliefs!**

## Why Diets Don't Work

My sister Sandi termed getting out of dieting and into a balanced healthy lifestyle as a legal U-turn. I love this. It is legal and it is your right! A total turnaround from all you have been taught is the way to a healthy, balanced weight. To help you choose to make a U-Turn in your lifestyle, I need to simplify why diets don't work. And why you don't need to follow another fad diet plan ever again once you follow the TEID Lifestyle.

The legal U-turn is a total change in your way of thinking. Remember when I said you are not at fault? Most people think life is about finding the next diet so they can look or feel like someone in an advertisement. At least they will feel this way for the first day or two. Then reality sets in. You find yourself unsatisfied, hungry, and craving certain foods—especially the ones you are told to avoid—while losing energy, having trouble thinking clearly, and just feeling crummy overall.

Almost every diet limits or eliminates fat, carbohydrates, or calories, but as we all know, there are a few popular diets in recent years that promote fat and reduced carbohydrates. I am not a big promoter of these diets, especially long-term. I support healthy balance, and I don't find cutting back on calories or carbohydrates to be balanced or a way of life you can maintain. I am not a promoter of filling my plate with just any fat. I am also not a promoter of counting calories.

# Chapter 4: Stop Blaming Yourself

When you are healthy and eating a balanced diet, your body controls how much fat it burns. Some diets promote forms of fasting, and I will give my opinion on fasting regarding healing and balance later in Chapter 6. The main point here is that maintaining an imbalance over a long period will have negative side effects on your health at some point. Not everyone is looking for the same lifestyle or process to reach their desired weight. I get that, and that's why there is a variety of people and various solutions. We are not all looking to be at our optimum weight and get our health balanced at the same time. What we know today and what we understand and learn tomorrow will hopefully advance.

We all know that most diets restrict calories, and as soon as you go back to eating a normal amount of calories, the weight gain begins again. And then there are the ever-so-common fat-free foods, which are heavily heaped into many diets. While eating fat-free you are most likely consuming processed foods and many chemically created sugar substitutes, which do not lead to a healthy balance. *Our bodies need fat.* Yes, they need fat; healthy fat. For many of you, this is a wonderful fact. No more eating foods that taste like cardboard! I will talk more about fats in Chapter 7.

Let's look at Webster's definition of the word diet:

> a. What is eaten and drunk habitually;
> b. a selected course of food, (verb) to cause to eat or drink, especially according to prescribed rules.[1]

For purposes of making a point here, when most people are asked what the word *diet* means to them, they elaborate on the second part of this definition. Often they expound on the rules in the form of restriction and/or weight loss. I have noticed that most of the time the word *diet* or *dieting* brings up the connotation of a specific diet or diet fad, as in fat-free diet, etc. I also often notice a feeling of defeat surface as they describe what diet means to them. Thus, I chose my company's name many years ago, "iDiet NO More," because I want to address the confusion and frustration most people live in while attempting to accomplish a task of weight loss and health through a variety of diet exercises. It seems that we have done a poor job of teaching what our bodies need to be healthy and stay at an optimum weight. And we have totally left out the fact that our bodies were created for health, not sickness or the weight challenges we observe today. My goal is to help unravel this confusion and enable people to turn their lives around and live a lifestyle based on nutrition and healthy balance. Not diet fads and misnomers.

Nutrition and nourishment and how diseases develop have everything to do with each other. The first signs we often notice from poor nutrition are obesity, being underweight, pain, illness, disease, dental problems, skin issues, a weak immune system, etc. Some people are dealing with what they inherited through their DNA, and I believe those things can be healed and turned around in time through implementing good nutrition and a

---

1. Webster's Collegiate Dictionary, s.v., "diet," (Sparingfield, Mass: G.C. Merriam Co., 1913).

balanced, healthy lifestyle. Therefore, the DNA we pass on in childbearing years can be a healthier DNA for our offspring.

I know all too well that many of you think I am talking to everyone else, that this turnaround couldn't be possible for you. You've tried so many diets and failed just as many times. Well, I am *especially* talking to you. I know the TEID Lifestyle will allow you to finally win and live a life of success. If you don't believe me, read Sandi's testimony one more time. You are the reason I am taking the time to write this book. Please don't give up! There's a way for you to win and make a simple legal U-turn in your life, and that can begin today. This turn will change your life and your future forever.

What iDiet NO More means to me is *never* going back to the yo-yo dieting lifestyle that so many live in. It means finding a way to simplify your life and live a healthy, balanced lifestyle that brings so many positive side effects: health, balance, and longevity are just a few examples.

Think about this for a minute. By taking this journey for yourself, you can in turn leave your loved ones or friends the testimony of a healthy, balanced lifestyle. Plus, the "how to do it" instructions will be played out in front of them. My family has caught on and they are enjoying the legacy they are building as they live a healthy, balanced lifestyle together. Can you imagine that? You now have the opportunity to pass on life—a life filled with quality and quantity, where families can be at their optimum weight and play together for many years into old age, all while their pain is being diminished or completely gone!

No more sitting on the sidelines, watching and wishing that you felt good enough about yourself or able to play too. It's time to get into the game of life if you feel left out. My husband and I love to celebrate life by having fun with our five grandchildren every time we get together. Life is too short to miss out on fun times and celebrations.

## A Key Reason You Can't Lose Weight

If you don't need to lose weight or you are not interested in it, please stay with me and read this chapter anyway. This chapter will clarify many of the false understandings you have been raised with regarding nutrition. And as the truth makes more sense to you, then the changes you are implementing will have greater value.

Our nation's national nutrition policy reaches into almost every American's life and has been taught to our doctors and dieticians for years. They have set the guidelines that all meal plans and feeding programs are based on, including meals in schools, hospitals, nursing homes, and homeless shelters and soup kitchens, to name a few. It is the policy that the health and wellness curriculum is based on in our schools.

# Chapter 4: Stop Blaming Yourself

I mentioned earlier that it is not your fault, and I will say it this way: Much of the teaching you received while growing up or in educational programs *are from misleading guidelines*. Most nutritional teachings have stemmed from the foundational food pyramid or food guide. This has changed slightly over the years; unfortunately, the guidelines do not recognize that various diagnoses, such as forms of diabetes, can be reversed with proper nutritional intake. Let me break this down for you and touch on some highlights over the years.

The USDA's food guidance chart began in 1916 with an attempt to show Americans how to select foods for their families that met bodily needs, with some discussion of measurement and defining protective foods.

In the 1940s, the update focused on showing what seven food groups we should choose from to receive nutrient adequacy. The seven categories were:

- Group 1 - Green and yellow vegetables (raw, cooked, frozen, or canned)
- Group 2 - Oranges, tomatoes, grapefruit, raw cabbage, and salads
- Group 3 - Potatoes, other vegetables, and fruits (raw, dried, cooked, frozen, or canned)
- Group 4 - Milk and milk products (fluid, evaporated, dried milk, or cheese)
- Group 5 - Meat, poultry, fish, or eggs (dried beans, peas, nuts, or peanut butter)
- Group 6 - Bread, flour, and cereals (natural whole-grain or enriched or restored)
- Group 7 - Butter and fortified margarine (with added vitamin A)

The number of servings was listed even though they did not say what a serving amount consisted of.

It is important to note here that the food they were selecting from had a completely different nutrient base than the food we choose from today. But the USDA guidelines most certainly gave Americans a place to begin.

From 1956 to the 1970s, the focus was on food for fitness, a daily food guide using the Basic Four. This group focused on goals for nutrient adequacy including specified amounts but did not give guidance on appropriate fats, sugars, and calorie intake. This group consisted of the milk group, meat group, vegetable and fruit group, bread and cereal group. This was the era I was raised in.

Then in 1979 after the development of the US dietary goals were released, they presented a hassle-free food group. This group consisted of the vegetable and fruit group, bread and cereal group, milk and cheese group, meat, poultry and bean group, with a focus on a fifth group to highlight the need to moderate intake of fats, sweets, and alcohol. Remember, fast-food restaurants had become more prevalent by this time.

## You Can Live Like This

In 1984 they changed it to a food wheel to simplify it even further. The five food groups and the amounts became the basis for the food guide pyramid. These groups were fruits, vegetables, fish-poultry-meat-eggs-nut/seeds, fats-sweets-alcohol, cheese-milk-yogurt, breads-grains-cereals. At this point, our nation began to experience a major increase in weight gain and obesity. A strong factor was the increase in grain consumption. During this time, eating out became more of a regular occurrence.

In 1992 the food pyramid guide was changed using consumer research to bring awareness to new food patterns. The pyramid illustration they used focused on concepts of variety, moderation, and proportion. The pyramid also was intended to illustrate a range for daily amounts of food across three calorie levels. It was demonstrated as such: the base of the pyramid consisted of breads-cereals-rice-pasta group (6-11 servings). The second level of the pyramid was the vegetable group (3-5 servings) and fruit group (2-4 servings). The third levels were shown as milk-yogurt-cheese (2-3 servings) and meat-poultry-fish-dry beans -eggs-nut group (2-3 servings). And at the tip of the pyramid were fats-oils-sweets (used sparingly).

In 2005 the name was changed to the MyPyramid Food Guidance System. This new system included daily amounts of food at twelve calorie levels. Their goal was to make a more simplified illustration. They added a band for oils and the concept of physical activity. In this illustration, they once again described the concept of variety, moderation, and proportion. The groups consisted of grains, vegetables, fruits, milk, and meat and beans. The pyramid illustration became vertical segments instead of horizontal segments and the width of the segments was meant to describe the amount in proportion to the day. And the concept of physical activity was demonstrated with a figure walking up a staircase on the left side of the pyramid.

In 2011 the title was changed to MyPlate. This change was intended to create a different shape to help grab the consumer's attention with a new visual cue. The illustration was a plate with a glass and a fork on a placemat. This icon served as a reminder for healthy eating, not necessarily intended to provide specific messages. And the word *my* was intended to continue the personalization approach from MyPyramid. The groups were identified as such: the glass is labeled dairy, the plate is broken into pie shapes and shows vegetables and fruits dividing the left side of the plate, with vegetables being a greater portion than fruits. The right side of the plate is grains and proteins, with grains having the greater portion.

Much of this has been an experiment on our nation's health. We are currently suffering severely from the unhealthy, low-fat diet that has been encouraged to combat the rise in obesity and diabetes. Unfortunately, I want to remind you that low-fat normally means high sugar. To understand the facts and see where we have come to, check out the link in the footnotes for the 2020-2025 guidelines and go to "Facts About Nutrition-Related

## CHAPTER 4: STOP BLAMING YOURSELF

Health Conditions in the United States."[2] You will see that our guidelines are not creating balance—but are creating many health issues that are causing serious concern.

## My Opinion of the Government Food Groups

*Today more than any time in the past, we lack knowledge about our food.* This might be difficult to believe because we have more information at our fingertips today than in any other era. What many people don't realize is our food today is extremely different from the food we consumed many years ago when compared in nutritional density. As we look at the United States in general, it is also obvious that we do not understand portion control, what foods contain the healthy nutrition our bodies so desperately need, and what foods are empty of nutrition but most likely are adding very unhealthy fats into our diet.

In general, most Americans don't value physical activity or understand how it aids their health. In short, most of us do not understand the importance of balance in our lives, or at least enough to make it a priority. Prioritizing balance will affect our health, our brains, and the longevity of our life.

When using the food guide, we have no explanation if it is a good guide for the areas that really matter. Let me explain.

## Vegetables

Vegetables have variety and how that variety needs to be eaten should be mentioned. Variety means a variety of vegetables that have a variety of nutrients. A variety of nutrients can often be identified by color, and this is especially true in vegetables.

Most of us will not take the time to click further on the link to see what other information is offered to us. There has been further explanation on each group. It is important to note that it is no longer a general rule of thumb that you eat so many servings; now there is a chart showing age with specific daily serving recommendations. In a general statement, it is stated that age, sex, or level of physical activity should be taken into consideration on servings.

## Fruits

Fruits vary, and it's helpful to understand which fruits are higher in sugar. You may have heard the terminology of high glycemic vs. low glycemic foods. This is especially valuable since our nation is dealing with an increase in diabetics. Diabetes is right up there in the top ten causes of death.

It also concerns me that fruit juice is equal to fruit in this category. You have to look hard to find apple juice made only from the juice of apples. Juice made from a concentrate with water, possibly with preservatives and sugars added, is, in no way, equal to a piece of

---

2. Dietary Guidelines for Americans, dietaryguidelines.gov, accessed January 7, 2022, https://www.dietaryguidelines.gov/sites/default/files/2021-03/Dietary_Guidelines_for_Americans-2020-2025.pdf

fruit. Most families today are consuming fruit juices that are loaded with unhealthy sugars and preservatives. When the food guide first began, it was not uncommon for families to squeeze their juice or for it to be fresh-squeezed when you purchased it at a produce market. This is not common for many of us today.

## Grains

Grains are identified as whole or refined (which may or may not be enriched). If the whole grain has been stripped but then enriched (meaning they have added nutrients back to the food following a process to strip it), they say it is good. I believe there is a large difference between the whole and refined/enriched grain. Once you begin the refining process, it strips the grain and then *may* add enrichment back into it. This is not the original nutrient content and fiber (previously stripped) that they are adding back in.

Consider a loaf of sliced white bread. First, the wheat is stripped of bran and fiber, and then it's pulverized into the finest of white flour. The baking process puffs it up into light, airy slices of bread. No wonder your stomach makes such quick work of it. A slice of white bread hits your bloodstream with the same jolt you'd get by eating a tablespoon of sugar right from the bowl!

Genuine 100-percent whole-wheat or whole-grain bread, on the other hand—the coarse, chewy kind with a thick crust and visible pieces of grain—puts your stomach to work. It, too, is made of wheat, but the grains haven't been processed to death. It contains starches, which are just chains of sugars, but they are bound up with fiber, so digestion takes longer. As a result, the sugars are released gradually into the bloodstream. If there's no sudden surge in blood sugar, your pancreas won't produce as much insulin and you won't get exaggerated hunger and cravings for more sugary and starchy carbohydrates.

I hesitate to get on one of my soapboxes here, but I am going to. Most bread is made with unhealthy fats/oils and have preservatives and other agents added that are not the best choice of fats available. Fortunately today, we have a few companies that have begun to focus on creating healthier alternatives.

## Protein

I find that the way protein is labeled is confusing to the general public. Protein is not a food group, it is a nutrient. Foods can contain the nutrient protein or not. To further make my point; there are several foods not listed in this food group, such as grains like quinoa, which are also considered protein-rich foods. On a personal note, I have a strong question about using soy (just any soy, not non-GMO soy) as if they are all equal. We all have our opinions on this.

Protein forms part of every cell in your body and is an important building block for your skin, muscles, bones, cartilage, and blood. In other words, your body requires protein for the structure, function, and regulation of the body's tissues and organs. Our

## Chapter 4: Stop Blaming Yourself

bodies cannot make protein, nor can they store protein. So this means getting enough protein in our diet is vital. Many fall short of consuming an adequate amount of protein daily. We need to meet our protein needs to keep our body functioning at its best.

**Milk**

Looking at their explanations of the milk group, you will find yogurt and fat-free yogurt is also listed. Fat-free yogurt or fat-free anything is generally filled with artificial sweeteners, which I recommend avoiding completely. The sugar count in regular yogurt can be mind-boggling if you serve this for your child's breakfast alone. Talk about a sugar crash once they arrive at school! And stripping the fat from any food product to eat fat-free has many, many consequences. I will spend more time talking about fat and fat-free later.

**Fat**

Lastly, fat is extremely important to the body's health. I am talking about healthy fat. One glance at the guidelines in the past reveals that there is no fat category and no mention of there being a difference between healthy and unhealthy fat. This should be a wake-up call! Heart disease and strokes are at the top of our nation's major killers, and unhealthy fats are one of the main culprits.

Remember when I said it is not your fault? This is the foundation from which you have been taught to eat and live to be healthy. But the problem is that you haven't been given enough information to choose how to fill your plate in a balanced manner unless nutrition is your passion or is part of your field of research, education, or work. I grew up watching these changes occur, and I would have missed it, too, if I hadn't focused on this subject.

I remember being taught health and nutrition in middle school. I took a class called home economics. This class was packed with nutrition and food preparation. I had a wonderful teacher. I took home economics for three years. That was long enough for most of this knowledge to become ingrained in me as natural concepts. Today I still practice many of the tips I learned back then.

The other challenge we all face is that there is such a barrage of information and even research out there, whether it be accurate or not, healthy or unhealthy, or just to make a buck. Sometimes the information and/or research comes from companies or people with their agendas, unbeknown to us. I know that it becomes overwhelming, to say the least. I am educated and I find it overwhelming to "find the meat while spitting out the bones."

We all live overly busy lifestyles, going to and fro and grabbing food wherever we can while hoping or trusting that it is good for our bodies. We think we know when we make a few poor choices but probably have not taken into consideration what might be in the food that we assume is a good choice, or how it was prepared or processed. Then the day comes when we get that wake-up call: health problems, obesity, pain, and the list could go on and on.

As you read on, I want to reiterate that my goal is to keep this simple, especially for people who have busy lives, even though this chapter may have seemed deep. Science is important, but that knowledge and understanding can come later.

The bottom line is this: if you never begin your journey to balance, *you will never get anywhere!* So let's get started and come back to fill in the blanks later. You will have more of an appetite for this knowledge after you start feeling better.

As I share with you what I see as balance, you can rest assured that if you follow these steps, your body can also get in balance and begin its repair. But if you choose not to make some simple changes to find balance, you will not begin your healing process or lose weight and keep it off. Nor will you rev up your metabolism, which is so important.

So the question is: are you ready? Do you choose life, health, balance, and longevity? Do you want to know how to get started? I have intentionally made this a *simple plan*.

*You can do this, and you will be so glad you did!* Let's go!

# Chapter 5

# FIRST STEPS

I cannot emphasize enough the value and importance of this chapter. If you skip it, you will not walk into the same success as those who implement these principles. I have simply stated the necessary steps to accomplish your optimal weight for life and live a healthy, balanced lifestyle.

## Make Yourself a Priority

If you are reading this book because you desire weight loss, please read this section as if you and I are the only ones in the room right now. I know how difficult it is to make yourself a priority, but it is truly the first step to your journey of success. You are worth it, and you will be amazed how you will draw attention from those around you as you begin your journey.

After just a few weeks you will feel a change and won't be able to hide the way your skin looks, the glow that you take on, and the smile and confidence you will walk in. There will be an extra kick to your step. Others will see this and ask what you are doing! And because you have more energy, sleep better, have improved mental clarity, and less pain (not to mention weight loss), you will be bubbling over to share how you're getting these results. If they know you and know your life story, they will most likely be attentive to what you share. This is a life-giving journey, so I hope you will share it!

We all know there are more naysayers than encouragers out there. So think of me as sitting with you right now, looking into your eyes and saying, "Put your blinders on; do not allow yourself to be distracted or discouraged. You are more valuable than you realize, and you can do this! Those who are trying to discourage you are jealous or just don't want to lose their eating buddy or party partner. This transition period will only last a season until your new habits become your lifestyle. This is your time! You will become stronger and stronger every week as your confidence grows and you feel better."

## You Can Live Like This

I know some are saying, "I feel good already." Yes, many of you do. But at the same time, you know there's room for improvement. Maybe you are not feeling as good as you could be, or you might not know what it feels like to feel really great because you are so familiar with feeling like you feel today. Maybe you have settled for having less energy with age or not sleeping as well as you used to. Regardless, permit yourself to make that legal U-turn today!

Listen to my sister, Sandi's, insight about making yourself a priority:

> No matter who you are or what your role is in life, what I am about to share is probably the hardest thing I had to conquer, and continue to conquer every day, on my journey to better health. Please don't think that I'm a selfish person for what I am going to share with you. I just know that learning this and implementing this priority as a daily focus, was a huge part of my success.
>
> I am a wife, mom, and grandma, and yes, I love to take care of my family in many ways, but for me to reach the success I so desired, I had to first take care of *me*! This meant focusing on myself every day. Some days were easier than others. I had to stay focused on meal planning, meal prepping, time for exercise, and time for learning and growing.
>
> There were days when I felt like a bobber on the end of a fishing pole and I would get too far away from where I needed to be and had to reel myself back in. It can happen easily. I now have a lifestyle that allows me to do this. I hope that as you implement this new way of life you, too, take time for yourself.
>
> A friend spoke these powerful words to me years ago: "If it is to be, it's up to *me*!" Unfortunately, it took me a long time to realize it, but I know it now—and that's what counts!

Making yourself a priority each day is a major key to your success. Remember that you're not alone. It's been a challenge for me too. I was raised to put others first, which is important, but I have learned that I must put myself first to achieve what I desire in my life. Once I learned how to do this, it didn't take time away from my day. It was just a new way of thinking about how I would prioritize my day.

Watching Sandi accomplish this simple, but at times challenging task has been beautiful. It has proved to make all the difference in her life. It is a foundational habit she and I formed for our daily balanced lifestyle. Sandi learned that she has what it takes to accomplish the greatest desires of her heart. And the best part of all has been to know that she feels so good about herself, along with watching her love living life to the fullest. Being a part of Sandi's journey has made it even more of a priority for me. It has created an excitement in me to share with the world—with those who are ready. Sandi and I both know that you have to be ready to take ownership of your health and life, and not be dependent on others to make it happen. Yes, Sandi, if it is to be, it's up to *me*!

# Chapter 5: First Steps

## Take Ownership

Taking ownership of my health and making my own decision regarding the path I would choose was the best way. This is what birthed the TEID Lifestyle. For Sandi and those whose testimonies you will read, the TEID Lifestyle was, and still is, their best option too. I have seen this ownership mindset help many people attain their goals. I encourage you to seek the same commitment for yourself. Use this book as your guidebook. It has been written in a simple and detailed format with you in mind. Don't wait for someone else to encourage you. You are your best cheerleader. Don't wait for someone else to join you or agree with you; take responsibility to prepare yourself, give your body the variety it needs, listen to your body, and set your own pace to Phase 3, the final phase. As I have already mentioned, don't get hung up on the little things. Keep moving forward. Believe in yourself. You have what you need inside of you and in this book. Consider yourself a winner!

## Variety Is Key

There are some thoughts in this chapter that may not flow as *proper* for many of you. Please keep an open mind. Move forward with me and remember that I plan to simplify this for you. Trying so many different diets kept many of you on the hamster wheel of counting calories, identifying every bite that goes into your mouth, and thinking about the next time you get to eat. Is that balance? Is that manageable for a lifetime? It isn't for me.

It is time for a little enjoyment of this thing called life and eating. The TEID Lifestyle is written as a guide for you. Use it! Let yourself dream about your life, where you want to go and what you want to do. Don't let the next meal consume your mindset. I want you to have freedom and not be stressed out when you walk into a restaurant or get together with friends for a meal. I want you to *know balance* and become empowered to make good choices. Enjoy this journey you are on! It's *your* journey and it's time to make the most of it.

Let's look at some key points so we can move forward to a new style of thinking and get you moving toward your success.

> **BALANCE + COLOR + VARIETY**
> **Will Be Your New Key to Success.**

Variety is very important. As you consume these forms of healthy nutrition, you will want to create a pattern of variation. Different foods contain different nutrients. This is very exciting and stimulating for your body. Okay, so that sounds crazy. But your cells are going to dance when they receive these nutrients. Parts of your body that have been almost asleep, so to speak, are going to wake up and take notice because the food is revving up and nourishing them.

## You Can Live Like This

For some, you don't even realize how badly you've been feeling. Once you experience this improvement, you will notice new life and new energy. It is a wonderful thing!

Some of you have learned to live with pain; you compensate for it and are vividly aware of it. When the pain lets up and begins to go away you may not sense it right away because you have learned to live that way. Most likely you weren't expecting your pain to disappear. Chronic pain comes from an injury or inflammation. Your brain remembers the pain and begins to create a process to deal with it. So when the pain goes away it is a delayed response to recognize that the pain is gone. Isn't it amazing that healthy nutrition helps reverse inflammation, which in turn causes your body's immune system to become stronger and bring balance and healing to itself? Our bodies are so incredible! The more you understand this the more you will appreciate all that you are.

We can't see what is going on under our skin, and we are all in our state of health. Therefore it is different for each of us; as to how long it will take for our healing to be noticed or for us to feel a change. But for most of us, we are so nutritionally depleted that just the least little bit of improvement toward balance will cause enough of a response in your body that you will notice. It might be even the slightest improvement, but it will be fuel to your journey.

As you focus on variety, begin to create a beautifully colored plate of food. Variety also equals a variety of colors, which is a result of the variety in nutrients. It is so simple. If you place a vegetable on your plate that is darkish green like broccoli, a piece of meat prepared in healthy fat covered in fresh herbs, and a bowl of mixed organic berries, you are becoming a food artist. *And it looks so yummy!* Just placing a sprig of your favorite herb like parsley on the side of the plate dresses it up and adds flavor too. I love using white plates at home. I also like rectangular or square plates for a fun addition. Get away from monotony. Let your creativity flow. This might be an area where you've not been creative in the past. Do not be afraid to try it. You can't fail, but you can have fun!

> **Some Helpful little Guidelines:**
> - The right portion of meat will fit perfectly in the palm of your hand when you hold your hand out palm up. That is generally equal to approximately three ounces of meat.
> - Your fist is usually equal to one cup.
> - The tip of your thumb (from the middle knuckle to the tip) is equal to approximately one teaspoon.
> - Growing up, you were told not to eat with your hands. Now, as an adult, I am telling you that you can eat with your hands!

These tips are just a place for you to begin. The real determining factor on portion size will come as you begin your journey. You don't need a food scale, but you will need a scale to weigh yourself on. We will discuss that in more depth in a few pages.

# Chapter 5: First Steps

## No More Counting Calories

I can't live on a calorie-counting diet. I can't live identifying every bite that goes into my mouth without thinking about food nonstop. And I don't eat boring food! If I don't like it I try to herb and spice it up, or cook it in healthy fat. When all else fails I dip it in a little coconut aminos (I will tell more on this in Chapter 9). I'm always finding a way to make my food have great flavor. I'm game to try everything. I love to cook!

I like to make a plate of food that looks like it came off the magazine cover from a famous chef's restaurant. I just happen to know one who has the perfect touch. One of my friends from high school, Joseph Keller, became a well-known and loved chef. My husband and I visited him in Nantucket one year for our fortieth anniversary. We spent every evening at his restaurant, "Company of the Cauldron." We were spoiled rotten. My husband wasn't sure about the trip when I planned it, but now he tells everyone about our trip—and especially the food! Joseph and his brother own several restaurants, and are the most enjoyable guys you will ever meet.

## Protein, Fat, and Carbohydrates

I meant it when I said I would not be teaching you how to count calories or balance your food by identifying it as a protein, fat, or carbohydrates. But I do categorize the foods in all the phases of the TEID Lifestyle for those of you who need that information. I know this goes against the grain for so many. That's okay; we all need to be free to pick what fits us best. So don't feel pressured if you just can't go here. I understand. You may not be ready.

Know that your friends may not tag along with you if you choose this. That's okay too. Maybe it's time to make new friends. Ha! I love friends and I don't think a healthy, balanced lifestyle is meant to be all about the food. Food is a huge part of it, but I don't want food to control my life—it should compliment and add enjoyment to my life.

This part of our journey is all about filling your plate with balance. You will choose healthy meat, a vegetable, and possibly a small amount of fruit (if you did not choose a starchy vegetable) and your choice of healthy fat. You will learn in Chapter 9 that having as many servings as you desire of healthy green leafy vegetables never gets old.

The more you learn to implement balance into your daily eating habits, the more familiar you will be with the added benefits. And the more you practice balance, the more you will see balance begin to pop up in other areas of your life too. Once you have established balance in various areas of your life, you are going to feel peace and contentment, not only with your life, but also with yourself and others—peace and contentment that you may not have ever experienced before. It's a beautiful side effect of a balanced healthy lifestyle, and it is fun! And let's not forget all of those new friends and new things going on in your life that you shied away from previously.

## You Can Live Like This

If you struggle with variety, now is the perfect time to try those items in the produce department or produce stand that you've never eaten before. Be brave, open-minded, and confident that you will enjoy it or that you might discover a new favorite. I've done this and now find it a wonderful part of my cooking experience. And, yes, it's okay to see yourself as a successful chef and let your creativity flow. This might well become a bucket list "check off" that you've never been brave enough to write down! All famous chefs started here too; experimenting and learning to be creative and unafraid to try new things.

I will mention this a few times throughout this book. I want you to find enjoyment in your food while nourishing your body properly as you begin to step out of the box you have lived in for too long. Eating variety adds diversity and newness to your day. It keeps your body thriving on a plethora of densely packed foods. This makes your body happy and healthy!

Using Phase 1 of the TEID Lifestyle will help you to begin with a focus on clean and healthy foods. As you advance through the phases of the TEID Lifestyle you will begin to add in new items. Once you are through all of the phases, you will be set for life. Then when vacation comes, just step back into a previous phase for a short period if you need help buckling back down. This isn't to say that vacation is a time to jump off the wagon of a healthy lifestyle, but if you are human and overindulge for a few days, you can get back on track right away while avoiding frustration and beating yourself up like you used to do. Those days are gone. You have a lifestyle that fits all situations, even when dining out or on vacation.

Some people never cook. I hope this will be an inspiration for you. If you never cook, give it a try. It could become a new hobby with friends. But if your daily routine is more trying and you hardly ever cook, you can still choose wisely. Print the guideline for each phase you are in and carry it with you. Use it as the guide it is meant to be to help you choose as wisely as you can. Take a minute and decide how to create the plate you might have created at home. If the meal comes with way too much food, just ask for the to-go box right away. Leave a good portion on the plate to eat and put the rest in the to-go box. Be a blessing by sharing the to-go portion with others if you know that eating that meal once was enough, especially if after you ate, it dawned on you that maybe that wasn't the best choice after all.

Notice that I never said you must clean your plate. You never have to clean your plate unless you *choose to*. You are in charge, and you will learn how to choose wisely. If you know you will dine out regularly, bring along little things that make choosing healthy meals fun, like your favorite herbs and seasonings, etc. If you know you're going to a restaurant that will tempt you to overindulge, plan to eat a little lighter during the day. I don't mean skipping meals; I mean choosing foods and snacks that yield the lighter side. Browse the menu before you arrive at the restaurant. This is a great opportunity to focus a little better and take your time to make the right choice. If you are able to look at the menu ahead of time, then don't look at it once you arrive at the restaurant. Just order what you already decided on. That is called taking charge and making a decision and holding to it. You will feel good about it then and later—I know!

# CHAPTER 5: FIRST STEPS

Here's a little trick when attending a party or gathering where there will be lots of party food or before going out to eat, just in case you have a longer wait time than expected. It can keep you from getting overly hungry before being served your scrumptious meal: Have a healthy snack like a cup of organic bone broth and a small apple or celery just before going out.

One of the most interesting things I know about the body is when you eat healthy foods, your body will crave healthy foods. When you eat junk food, your body craves junk food. It's a blessing in disguise. If we choose wisely and listen to our bodies, they will usually guide us. Stepping into this new lifestyle is a step up in so many ways.

## Listen to Your Body

When Bradley, our firstborn, was very young and too small to tell me why he felt bad, I remember visiting his pediatrician. I fully expected the doctor to tell me what he thought he was dealing with. After sharing why I had made the appointment, I was surprised when the doctor turned and looked at me and asked, "What do *you* think is going on?"

I looked back at him and replied, "What do *I* think?"

He said, "Yes, I have learned over my many years of practice not to go down a rabbit trail when I have the best source to give me an accurate starting point."

I remember being slow to respond because I was surprised at his interest in my gut feeling. I learned that day that as the mom, I could trust my inner instinct when it came to my kids.

My baby sister, Gina, calls this "trusting your knower." When her kids were growing up she told them when situations arise, just trust their knower. You know, it's that feeling deep inside of you. Generally, you will feel at peace when you trust your knower. And then she said, "If you don't feel at peace, don't go there! At least until you give further evaluation or consideration."

Good advice, Gina! That advice continues to work as we have gotten older. I might joke that I taught my sisters everything they know, being the oldest, but we learn from each other. Just like we learn from our boys and their families, especially our grandchildren. They keep us on our toes.

Taking Gina's advice a step further, I want to encourage you to "trust your knower" when it comes to your body, and tell you to listen to what your body is trying to tell you. Countless numbers of people run to a doctor or therapist for their opinion. Please let me say that I am not putting anyone or any professional down or that you should not consult them. But many times if you listen to your body, you will have an idea of what is going on under your skin. It may not come right away, but as you begin to pay attention and follow the symptoms, you will start to have some insight into the root issues. As the pediatrician said, at least it can keep you from running down a rabbit trail, and give you an idea of where to begin—at your diet, exercise, sleep pattern, etc.

The key to my healing came from listening to my body. I was making great progress when the doctor told me to take what I had learned and apply it. She said that I knew my body, I knew about nutrition, and if I began with a little elimination and experimentation, I would find more answers.

We lived a long distance from her office, so this was her way of helping me to help and trust myself. She was always only a call away. She mentioned that from her experience it was most likely going to involve gluten. We discussed how gluten today is not what it was when I was younger and therefore, even though I tolerated it then, maybe some current changes in the growing and harvesting of gluten were affecting me now, as it has many others. This made a lot of sense, and I left her office that day in December excited about the journey my husband and I were going to embrace. We jumped in with both feet and never looked back. My sister, Sandi, got excited that day too and, as you now know, came along with us on our journey. She began to learn to listen to her body too.

It became obvious that my gut had been suffering to some degree from foods I was not tolerating well. I wrote every single bite down to help identify which food or foods were involved. As you begin to prepare to begin Phase 1 of the TEID Lifestyle, keep a journal and make notes. We will talk about these points again further on, but I want to mention them now because they play a vital role as you listen to your body.

**You might have a few pages in your journal that look like this:**

- A menu for the day or the week
- A grocery list
- What I ate today, include times and foods (all ingredients)
- Body weight: record it daily
- Foods my body may not be excited about (date, food, and possible response)

When I began my journey, my body was not happy with garlic, a common item that I had been eating forever but didn't realize that my body wasn't responding to it well. I dealt with symptoms that were not very pleasant. It wasn't until I wrote it all down and listened to my body that I put two and two together. You will make the connections, too, as you journal.

## The Scale Is Your Friend

For most of us, the scale has been our enemy. It shows us the truth and what we don't want to see or deal with. But in the TEID experience, the scale will become your friend, almost like a guide. Yes, it still reveals the truth of the choices you made the day before, but now you can use this to your advantage. I want to encourage you to weigh yourself each morning. I have done this for as long as I can remember. Always record your weight and the date. I have a small, hardbound lined journal that measures four by six inches. It is lime green and has these words written on the front: "Ooh la la." I love it! This works for me, and I am going to have fun doing this. Come on, if we can't find the fun in the simple things we will miss it in the big things!

## Chapter 5: First Steps

I don't know a single woman who would weigh in the morning before going to the bathroom. Right? I like to weigh in the morning after that visit. On a side note without getting too personal, if I'm struggling to have daily bowel movements I know I probably need to balance out my hydration, fats, and fiber (vegetables and fruit) a little better.

### Record Your Weight Daily

So record your weight with the date every morning in your journal. I make a note if I'm not at home. That information reminds me that I was using an unfamiliar scale to account for any change that may have taken place in my weight that day.

I normally have breakfast next. I almost always have a protein shake and do my morning reading and planning to get my mind ready for the day. Then, when I have time to focus, I evaluate by looking at yesterday's food journal against my weight today. Did I have an incremental gain or loss of weight? At first this may seem like a task, but trust me, soon it will be a delight.

For someone trying to lose weight, a gain tells you that you didn't have a balance of nutrients, hydration, and/or portion size. A loss tells you that you did a good job of balancing. For the first week or two there may be some fluctuation. You need to give yourself space for this learning curve. Give yourself some grace. I mentioned before that this is not a diet that you will conquer, lose weight, and then eventually gain it all back. *This is a lifestyle.* A new lifestyle is something you will get stronger with, more confident in, and more comfortable with every single day as you diligently pursue the TEID Lifestyle.

If I see a gain, I examine my journal and see where I could improve my portion size or the balance of fruit and/or vegetables and the amount of fat that was included. You will begin to have a real handle on this within the first week. But don't beat yourself up if it takes longer. Spend that energy to become more creative with your next meal plans. This is a great time to bring a little exercise, like walking, into the picture. Keep your exercise light during the first two weeks, then increase as you get more balanced in your meal planning and see some results.

### Notes about Journaling Meals and Snacks:

- This can be in a regular spiral notebook or whatever form of notebook you like.
- Place the date at the top of each page.
- Each day gets its own page or two if it's a smaller notebook.
- Record the time for each entry.
- Record everything you eat or drink, the quantities, and the ingredients that go into the preparation of the meal. A measure can be used like the fist or a cup to remind yourself of the amount. Remember the guidelines in this chapter. This guide is going to help you now to gauge the amount of food placed on your plate.
- Do not eat the same foods over and over. Remember the importance of keeping variety.

# Chapter 6

# BALANCE

Many people today live in the hustle and bustle of life, and balance is not even a consideration. They don't know what balance looks like. As you begin to incorporate healthy balance into your eating habits, it will start to spill over into many areas of your life. This is a good thing! Healthy balance shows up in your blood work. Balance shows up in your attitude. Balance is reflected in your work. Balance comes out in your play.

Following the TEID Lifestyle is about balance and it is going to help you to live in balance, thereby improving your overall health and mindset about everything.

## What Healthy Balance Looks Like

Healthy eating involves eating a variety of natural foods that give you the nutrients you need to maintain your health, feel good, and have energy. These nutrients include proteins, fats, carbohydrates, water, vitamins, and minerals.

Unhealthy eating includes foods that are low in nutrients, high in empty calories, high in sugars, high in unhealthy fats, high in unnatural preservatives and artificial sweeteners. Good nutrition is an important part of leading a healthy lifestyle, but it is not all of it.

When I talk about balance in this book, I am referring to six forms of balance that should all work together:

- Nutrition
- Hydration
- Exercise
- Sleep
- Stress
- Spiritual

## You Can Live Like This

I believe these six parts of balance all work together in your body to create your balanced health or lack of it. I will touch on each of these. So often we ignore the symptoms our body is trying to give us until we have that wake-up call in our health or begin to have pain. Some are not lucky enough to have this opportunity. Since you are reading this book, you are one of the blessed ones and can take this information and apply it as you choose.

**Nutrition**

Our bodies are living vessels. They need and thrive on good nutrition to stay alive and in good health. Without it, they get sick and diseased and/or become out of balance with a poor metabolism and undesired weight gain or loss. Not to mention the aging that can take place. With this in mind, you now know how important it is to understand good nutrition.

Unfortunately, today it's not as easy as it was fifty years ago to find foods filled to the brim with nutrients, *but it is possible*. You have to educate yourself and make good choices. One of my goals is to help you rev up your engine with nutrition and get your metabolism working for you, not against you, so that you can achieve your optimum weight and feel good while doing it. I know I sound like a broken record, but I want you to begin to believe this is possible for you.

Remember that supplementation has its place, but never as a substitute for proper nutrition. It is just what the name suggests: a supplement—an addition to, an extra element of (support). Many supplements are dependent on proper nutrition being in place to help break down and absorb the ingredients of the supplement to yield beneficial effects to your body.

And, yes, I want to keep it simple for you so wherever you're at—be it eating at home, sitting at your desk with your sack lunch, or in a restaurant—you can choose the best available balanced nutrition. You can do this with a few basic and simple guidelines in place. Of course, this will always include a variety of nutrients and colors to achieve well-balanced nutrition.

To the best of your ability, always avoid processed and refined foods. This is the beginning of leading a healthy, balanced lifestyle combined with the items I mentioned above to achieve and maintain a healthy weight and reduce your risk of chronic diseases; like heart disease, diabetes, and cancer. This is all to promote your overall health. It's true! *A happy healthy body leads to a happier you.*

**Hydration**

Hydration is very important. We have all heard that drinking water is important, but many don't realize why it is so valuable. Water is the most important nutrient our bodies depend on to survive. Every cell, tissue, and organ in your body needs water to work properly. Your body uses water to maintain its temperature, remove waste, lubricate its joints, cleanse the

## Chapter 6: Balance

body from toxins, maintain healthy skin, hair, and organs, produce digestive enzymes, and help your body absorb essential vitamins, minerals, and natural sugars.

Since water is so important to our bodies I want to share some thoughts about how you can naturally get healthy water. I know most of you buy bottled water to drink on the go or maybe even to consume at home. If you do, glass bottles are always the best choice. But if you want to save money and create your water at home and know what you are drinking, I recommend you buy a Berkey countertop water filter system. They have stainless steel chambers, and the only maintenance is changing the filter once a year. We have used this system for so many years. We have even carried our smaller system with us while traveling. We especially love using it when all we have available to us is city water. These systems come in various sizes and the Berkey filters are reported to remove bacteria, chloramine, chromium 6, fluoride, lead, and pharmaceuticals. Once the water passes through the filters, we just fill the glass bottle, stick it in the refrigerator or our carry-along stainless steel cup, and go. We make our ice from this water too.

We lose water through our breath, perspiration, urine, and bowel movements every day. So it needs to be replenished daily by consuming beverages and foods that contain water.

*So how much fluid does the average, healthy adult living in a temperate climate need?*

So you've probably heard the advice to drink eight glasses of water a day. That's easy to remember, and it's a reasonable goal.

Most healthy people can stay hydrated by drinking water and other fluids whenever they feel thirsty. For some people, fewer than eight glasses a day might be enough. But other people might need more.

You might need to modify your total fluid intake based on several factors:

- Exercise: If you do any activity that makes you sweat, you need to drink extra water to cover the fluid loss. It's important to drink water before, during, and after a workout.
- Environment: Hot or humid weather can make you sweat and requires additional fluid. Dehydration also can occur at high altitudes.
- Overall health: Your body loses fluids when you have a fever, vomiting, or diarrhea. Drink more water or follow a doctor's recommendation to drink oral rehydration solutions. Other conditions that might require increased fluid intake include bladder infections and urinary tract stones.
- Pregnancy and breastfeeding: If you're pregnant or breastfeeding, you may need additional fluids to stay hydrated.

# You Can Live Like This

**Exercise**

This is not a book about exercise, but I cannot impress enough the importance of exercise. As is always first and foremost, if you are under the care of a health care practitioner, it is wise to allow them to make personal exercise suggestions for you. Exercise affects the whole body. Learning how to improve nutrition and incorporate exercise to stay healthy and in balance helps you learn simple ways to improve your heart health. Additionally, exercise helps build collateral circulation to support good heart health as you get older. There are many great articles and books on exercise. I might write more about this later, but in this book I just want to encourage you to begin.

If you currently do not exercise, start slowly. Walking is a great place to begin. As you get started, increase your speed after a few minutes and swing your arms to a level you can tolerate. Just swinging your arms as you walk increases your cardiovascular workout. You can't go from sitting on the sofa to running a marathon in a week or two; that's not balanced or possible without injuring yourself. Begin by working up to a brisk (arm swinging) power walk multiple times a week and then move on to a faster speed, longer distance, then add other forms of exercise as your body is ready for it and as your doctor encourages you.

*You should not endure exercise; you should enjoy it.* This is very important! With that said, it may take a little effort, but figure out what type of exercise you enjoy. Each person is different and so are their bodies. Some enjoy running, while others enjoy swimming. Some enjoy tennis, while others enjoy golf. Whatever you like, that is the best place to begin. Since you are reading this book and beginning to follow a balanced plan, please keep an open mind. It will encourage your growth toward your goal.

With exercise, it helps to change it up sometimes. Just like we don't want to eat the same food over and over, we want to have a variety of nutrients to feed our bodies a well-balanced diet. It is the same with working out—we don't want to do the same exercise over and over. Use various muscles and do various levels of exercise regularly. In other words, rotate what you do on different days of the week.

If you are an avid exerciser, please keep in mind that if your nutrition, hydration, and sleep are not balanced, you may be increasing inflammation. This can occur as a result of exercising too much without properly feeding your body before workouts and giving rest to your cells and muscles. Even exercise is to be kept in balance. Nutrition feeds your body at a cellular level. Your body knows how to get nutrition delivered to the organs, nerves, muscles, and skin. If you are an avid exerciser but do not focus on nutrition, you could be doing damage. Even though you may feel great now, one day there is a chance it could surface. You may also make yourself more susceptible to injury, which is a bad word for any athlete.

# Chapter 6: Balance

If you are limited physically, you're not alone. Begin by talking to your doctor and support system. There is most likely something you can do to begin. If you're in physical therapy at this time, ask for a plan that you can build on as you are ready for more. If you have pain when you exercise, determine what your limit is, act accordingly, and take it slowly. Your goal is not to cause more injury.

If you can't walk, maybe you could begin by flexing and extending your feet where you sit. Remember, some activity is better than no activity. Start where you are able and increase your exercise from there. It's about you. Not about what others can do or are doing. Take time to feel good about yourself. Be proud, even if you are only making small accomplishments—they are still accomplishments!

**Exercise and BMI**

Exercise can help improve your BMI (body mass index). BMI is a measure of body fat based on your weight to your height, and applies to most adult men and women age twenty and over. BMI is used as a screening tool to indicate whether a person is underweight, overweight, obese, or a healthy weight for their height. This is not considered by many to be accurate enough to use as a diagnostic tool. BMI does not measure body fat directly.

If a person's BMI is out of the healthy BMI range, their health risks may increase significantly. BMI can be measured by a BMI calculator or a BMI chart. BMI is your weight (in kilograms) over your height squared (in meters). It is quite easy to do an Internet search for a BMI calculator. Enter your height and weight into the calculator to determine your BMI. BMI charts are quite readily available online too.

Remember that it is just a tool. Some feel there is much room for error in this calculation, due to variation in body frame size, muscle mass, and/or bone density, to name a few. If you can identify that spare tire around your middle, it would be easy to assume that your BMI is still needing a little work. Therefore, my encouragement to you is to work to achieve an optimum weight, healthy, balanced lifestyle with regular exercise and good nutrition as a starting place. It is only natural that your BMI will improve as you move forward to achieve these goals, and all of your efforts will all work together to make a healthier more balanced you.

**Sleep**

Sleep plays a very large part in maintaining balance; probably a bigger role than most of us realize. Some can sleep a good eleven hours a night, while others struggle to sleep two to three hours. If you need more sleep, most likely improving your nutrition and finding balance in other areas of your life will also improve your sleep.

I want to encourage you in this area so much because I spent many segments of my life struggling to sleep well. I have a high energy level and just never seemed to require a lot of sleep. But the fact is that our bodies need rest and sleep to repair. So sleep is a priority, especially if you are an avid exerciser. I encourage you to keep in mind that the averages shown below in the chart of recommendations are a good balance to shoot for. In other words, the happy medium between the high and low recommendation for a nightly goal is what I would encourage you to shoot for. Too little sleep tends to impact inflammation, and too much sleep can carry inflammatory factors. I think most of you will find this recommendation chart interesting and helpful.

**National Sleep Foundation's Sleep Duration Recommendations:**

| Age | Age Range | Recommended |
| --- | --- | --- |
| Newborns | *0-3 months* | 14 to 17 hours |
| Infants | *4-11 months* | 12 to 15 hours |
| Toddlers | *1-2 years* | 11 to 14 hours |
| Preschoolers | *3-5 years* | 10 to 13 hours |
| School-aged Children | *6-13 years* | 9 to 11 hours |
| Teenagers | *14-17 years* | 8 to 10 hours |
| Young Adults | *18-25 years* | 7 to 9 hours |
| Adults | *26-64 years* | 7 to 9 hours |
| Older Adults | *≥ 65 years* | 7 to 8 hours[3] |

The recommendations result from multiple rounds of consensus voting after a comprehensive review of published scientific studies on sleep and health. The expert panel included six sleep experts and experts from the American Association of Anatomists (experts on anatomy) and the American Academy of Pediatrics.

## Help Yourself Sleep Better

I want to encourage those who don't sleep well to be willing to try a few new things that could help.

- Begin a bedtime ritual that works best for you. In other words, figure out what works and retrain yourself to do it.
- Do NOT have any electronics in your room.
- Lights out. Darkness helps.
- Try a warm bath before bedtime with your favorite essential oil for relaxation or using a diffuser to fill your room with a relaxing essential oil fragrance. If you don't desire either of those, then just dab a little essential oil on a tissue and place it under your pillow. I mix almond seed oil with lavender essential oil in a mister that I spray on my

---

3. Eric Suni, "How Much Sleep Do We Really Need?" The Sleep Foundation website, accessed March 7, 2022, https://sleepfoundation.org/press-release/national-sleep-foundation-recommends-new-sleep-times/page/0/1

# Chapter 6: Balance

chest. I also use a diffuser in my home and bedroom with various oils; lavender is my favorite go-to for relaxation along with a drop of peppermint. These help me to set the scene for relaxation. It was trial and error for me to determine which oils helped me. Be willing to experiment. Your body will love you for it.

- Meditation. I love to meditate on a verse in Psalms, as it brings me such peace. If I wake in the middle of the night and can't fall back asleep easily, I go back and recall the verse I meditated on before bedtime. I'm usually asleep before I get through that thought.
- Magnesium supplementation helps, especially if I had a good bit of exercise that day.
- A walk or stretching with deep breathing before or combined with meditation can be helpful. Try ten minutes of relaxing stretches mixed with relaxing instrumental music. I also like soothing piano music to create a peaceful atmosphere.
- Drink fewer fluids after dinner if you get up during the night a lot. If it's not an issue, a warm small cup of herbal caffeine-free tea for relaxation might be helpful. I normally don't drink any caffeine after two p.m. to avoid the side effects later.
- Exercise helps me prepare for sleep if I do it in the evening. I think it is because of my high energy. For others, it may be a stimulant. Do what is best for you—figuring out your body's needs is so helpful. Listen to your body; it will show you what it does and doesn't like!
- If you have a lot on your mind, take the time to clear it out. I can't emphasize this enough. If I don't do this, it comes back to me in the middle of the night. And the middle of the night is *totally* when I don't want to deal with it. Whether you need to pray over someone or something, do it or write it down so you can deal with it in the morning. Just don't muddle over it. Place a notepad and pen next to your nightstand. Once you write it down you can forget it. We have all experienced a molehill growing into a mountain in the middle of the night. You can come back to it in the morning when the sun comes up and you are rested and fresh. Things usually look better in the daylight. If you need to take time to work through some idea or thought that has been pestering you all day, jot a few notes to remind yourself, or take a minute and deal with it. The more you practice this, the simpler and more routine it becomes. Several books have well documented that *it's all small stuff anyway*. So give thanks for your day. Gratitude and thankfulness are open doors to welcome a peaceful sleep.
- Tell yourself you will not be dependent on sleeping aids, that you can do this. Maybe you need to do a gradual decrease with your doctor's direction instead of just stopping them cold turkey. Make up your mind to conquer the things you want to, and hold yourself to your decisions. Take time to form good sleeping habits, and you won't have to bounce from doctor to doctor to try new sleeping aids. If you temporarily supplement with some medications, don't beat yourself up, but don't lose sight of your goals and what you know you can do that will make a difference.

- Make sure your bedroom and bed are super-inviting, comfy, and are at the right temperature. Most of us sleep best in a cooler environment. It might help to organize your bedroom; have less clutter or try going minimalist in your bedroom. Some find that just the simple act of making their beds in the morning helps them feel happier and more welcomed to their sleep space at night. Make sure your mattress and pillow are to your liking, even the linens. Try changing the position you sleep in too.
- Reading is restful and could definitely put you to sleep, but probably not on your phone, tablet, or device. Or it could be stimulating for some.
- Limit alcohol right before bedtime. Even though it seems to relax you then, it can alter your sleep patterns and the quality of your sleep. When the alcohol level in your body drops a few hours later, it can wake you up and cause feelings of agitation, making it difficult to sleep peacefully for the rest of the night.
- Eat lightly before bedtime, especially avoiding foods that might cause you indigestion. On the flip side, don't go to bed hungry. Have a healthy, light snack when needed.
- Set a schedule. Form new sleeping habits by going to bed at a certain time, as well as waking up at a planned time. You will be amazed how your body adapts and obeys.
- Don't take long afternoon naps. Resting and getting your second wind is a little different than getting a good sleep in the middle of the day. I'm not talking about naps that don't interfere with your sleep. Some have a routine, and it includes catching a nap. If you need more rest, a nap may be beneficial—especially if you're ill or in recovery.
- Adding exercise to your daily regimen helps with all kinds of things that may interfere with your sleep, like anxiety and depression. Still, it also provides specific physiological boosts to sleep. Exercise strengthens circadian rhythms and may stimulate longer periods of slow-wave sleep, the deepest and most restorative phase of sleep.
- Keep the environment quiet. Using a white noise machine has become very popular for use with babies and children and can help adults mask all that ambient sound, along with sudden noises like a door closing, especially when traveling or not in your normal environment. A fan or air purifier can work well too. Sometimes, soft, slow instrumental music is my go-to, especially when I am in a hotel. It creates a sense of homey comfort along with the essential oils in my mini travel diffuser.

**Stress**

Here is one thing we all have in common—stress. I have yet to meet a person who has never experienced stress. I am only going to take time here to make a recommendation to find what works for you. There are countless self-help books available on how to help yourself to become less stressed. I have tried many things over my lifetime, and the ones that have brought me the most success are:

- Exercise of choice, including some stretching and deep breathing.

# Chapter 6: Balance

- Prayer, praise, being grateful, despite my apparent circumstances (which might be tainted due to lack of sleep or my schedule being overfull), and reading scripture, especially a Psalm and Proverbs.
- Remember that almost everything I am stressing over is just small stuff; it is not life or death. That helps me. It is common that when I wake in the morning with daylight shining on the scene, what seemed quite a big deal last night now looks silly, and I wonder how it could have even stolen one minute of my sleep and peace the night before.
- Deep breathing, stretching, and just meditating and giving it to God often works in the Let Go and Let God mindset.
- Maintaining your spiritual balance.
- Set boundaries. Not everyone has the right to pour into your life, especially those who may dump. In other words, they bring problems but are not seeking solutions. They want someone to fix things for them. Often they tend to see the cup half empty instead of half full. This yields to a negative mindset and imbalance in their life that can spill over into your life if you are too close. Don't make their issues your issues.

I have come to realize over the years that when I'm tired, everything seems more challenging to handle. All of my problems seem like a giant when I'm exhausted, so I do my best at night to create a good environment for proper rest for myself. It's a priority for me to stay on schedule and get the number of hours of sleep I need to function. I feel more balanced, happier, and I can handle life's ups and downs so much better when I am rested and seeing things from the proper perspective.

**Spiritual**

Since I have the pen, these are coming from my personal beliefs. My beliefs are not in any way intended to make you feel intimidated or in lack—just the opposite. If you don't have an understanding of who you were created by and who you were created to be, then I encourage you to get answers to these questions and to know your true identity. Some have a belief system already in place, maybe something that was passed down to you from your family or friends.

I want to encourage you during this journey to begin to solidify who you are and what your beliefs are. Maybe what was passed down to you doesn't feel like your own belief. Or maybe you have grown in a different direction from the former beliefs you were handed. As we talk about the human body, I will often mention what it is capable of doing, for example, healing itself with proper nutrition. I want to give you the opportunity, too, if you so desire, to see what a powerful vessel your body truly is.

For me, the spiritual aspect of who I am ties these six forms of balance all together for my greater benefit. It's like the cement that holds me together and in balance. I believe science has given us great insight into the incredible ways of the human body. Yet we are still learning and discovering all God has for us. He made His creation to eat food to sustain the physical body, including keeping it free from sickness and disease. I believe we are also supposed to eat spiritual food to sustain our spiritual person. I am already looking forward to finishing this book and revealing my second book, which will focus on spiritual balance and knowing who you were created to be. This has been life changing for me, and I know it will bless those who are hungry to know more. It will give insight into the power available to live an abundant, balanced lifestyle.

## A Healthy Balance Can Produce Healing

This chapter is for those seeking further understanding, or are wondering if a healthy balance can produce healing to improve health, weight loss, or want to get pain under control. The answer to this question is a firm "Yes!" Balance can produce healing. It doesn't happen overnight; it took many years to arrive where you are today, but you will be surprised how quickly your body will respond to healthy, balanced nutrition. It can be shocking if you haven't experienced this before. So many people have told me, "I can't believe after just a week or two that I feel better!" Even a slight improvement is a step toward better health.

Your body spent years trying to figure out what to do with that unhealthy processed food, and it will be so happy to receive some real nutrients from your food choices now. The human body was created to process food and put the nutrients in the food to work. These nutrients help achieve balance and health. Now that you are doing an about-turn, and striving to give balance to your body, it will jump to attention and go beyond anything you can imagine to thank you and begin to make good use of what you are feeding it. So many have felt that making this little U-turn has been life-changing for them.

To state it simply, you feed your body healthy, balanced nutrients (aka real nutrient-dense food), and the nutrients are processed and arrive at the cellular level to feed living cells in your body. Good nutrition brings a balance at this cellular level by helping inflamation decrease. This leads to many things: detoxification, healthier organs and systems, less inflammation, balanced hormone production, your metabolism waking up and going to work for you, improved mental clarity, sleeping better, and an overall feeling of balance, peace, and harmony within your body.

I talked earlier about maintaining balance, and I addressed six specific areas that balance should be found in: nutrition, hydration, sleep, stress, exercise, and spirituality. One indirectly affects the other. The more attention you give to overall balance, the better and more lasting lifelong results you will receive.

## Balance Means Eating Regularly

Earlier I mentioned that you would not deal with hunger like most diets you have previously endured. That's because on the TEID Lifestyle, you will eat every three hours. By doing this, you supply your body with nutrients and maintain a balanced blood sugar

# Chapter 6: Balance

level. When your blood sugar is balanced, you'll likely feel energetic, happy, productive, and will sleep well. I have heard countless ugly dieting testimonies of people being "hangry" (bad-tempered or irritable as a result of hunger). Who hasn't experienced that at one time or another? Do you remember trying to starve or to stretch yourself between non-fat meals to non-fat snacks, and trying to think clearly and keep functioning? When you follow the TEID Lifestyle, you will not be hangry!

I want you to begin to see an imaginary plate divided into three sections. Picture the sections filled like this: ⅓ meat, ⅓ vegetables/fruit, ⅓ fat. The fat can be healthy oils you prepared the meat or vegetables in, or it can be fat like avocado. Even though you envision a plate divided into thirds, there, most likely, will not be a clear division between each section when the meal is served. The fats will be blended with the other foods, resulting in a balanced meal on your plate.

Chapter 10 will give you a seven-day sample meals/snacks to get you started. Here is a sample schedule for meals and snack times to clarify the timing I mentioned above:

>   6:30 a.m. - Breakfast
>   9:30 a.m. - Snack
>   12:30 p.m. - Lunch
>   3:30 p.m. - Snack
>   6:30 p.m. - Dinner
>   9:00-9:30 p.m. - Bedtime Snack

## Fasting

Notice that approximately between 9:30 p.m. and 6:30 a.m., you are fasting. Other than this, you will not be fasting until you complete Reintroduction and Phase 3, and then you can add it in at your discretion. When beginning Phase 1 and even in Phase 2, fasting would not bring balance and would slow down your metabolism. In Chapter 2, I spoke about revving up your metabolism. Additionally, we are working to decrease inflammation.

I believe fasting will increase inflammation at this early stage, especially if it's already an issue. We are striving to bring healing by decreasing the current inflammation. I will discuss fasting more in-depth and from a few different angles in the next book.

## What about Supplements?

Our bodies look for nutrition for survival, and most of us are feeding them sugars, fillers, preservatives, and unhealthy fats—and then we top that off with a handful of supplements, which are often even more of the same. Try to picture this with me: your bodies cells are looking at that *so-called food* and saying, "What is that? What do I do with it? Where is the real stuff?"

## You Can Live Like This

Many people eat poorly and follow it down with a handful of any type of over-the-counter supplements. Meanwhile, they think they are filling in the gap to better health while consciously eating poorly. I am not a big promoter of supplements just to override poor nutrition.

Today supplementation is probably more important than it has ever been. And our world is full of supplement companies touting to be the best, but in all honesty, very few are. When you are attempting to get back to balance—or for some, to get into balance for the first time—you most likely will need to support different parts of your body with various supplements. Of course, this is in addition to good nutrition from the foods you eat, which is always a priority. As I mentioned earlier, our food today does not have the nutritional density that foods fifty years ago had. I also feel that most people today are living under a much higher stress level. So I do encourage good supplementation more often now than I would have even five or ten years ago.

Getting healthy nutrition and supporting your body to digest and use these nutrients is an asset as you transition to balance. So the first areas to glean support are pre-and/or probiotics, digestive enzymes, and multivitamins. This will be based on an individual evaluation because, in most cases, not one supplement fixes all. Some of you are dealing with inflammation, while others digestive issues, and others, total gut imbalance. Any of these can lead to your body's inadequacy to absorb the nutrients. Not to mention that if you're not feeling good, you most likely can't lose weight, you will have lack of energy, a foggy brain, or serious chronic health problems. So this can clearly become a much bigger issue than many of us have understood.

As we age, some of these supplements may be more important to maintain regularly than others that might be useful for a season of repair and balance. Various health conditions, stress levels, or workout routines are also determining factors in the needs of our body.

I want to encourage you to look for *whole food supplements* and discover with your health-care professional or for yourself which ones are most easily absorbed and will be more fully used by your body. All supplements are *not* created equally. You will quickly learn this for yourself as you begin to journey and research into the different ways supplements can be made.

This particular writing intends to address healthy nutrition and balance and to begin to open your mind to the need for healthy supplementation along with proper nutrition, *not in place of it*.

My favorite whole food supplement company is Optimal Health Systems. If you are interested in reading about their products, you can visit this link:

**OptimalHealthSystems.com/#code=OHSBRYNTESON**

If you need assistance, please contact me through my website - iDietNoMore.com.

# Chapter 7

# INFLAMMATION

Before we delve into the TEID Lifestyle, I want to share with you what is going on in our bodies at a cellular level as close to layman's terms as possible. Cellular inflammation is the type of inflammation that is below the perception of pain. It disrupts hormonal signaling at the cellular levels that leads to increased fat accumulation, acceleration of the development of chronic disease, and decreased physical performance. In other words, you can't feel cellular inflammation as it begins. It is the initiating cause of chronic disease because it disrupts hormonal signaling networks throughout the body. Inflammation sometimes persists for a long time, even without an infection or injury. This is called chronic inflammation. This long-term inflammation can contribute to almost every chronic illness, including heart disease and cancer.

I'm often asked if there's a blood test to measure inflammation in our bodies. Yes, there is. The blood test is called CRP (C-reactive protein). Most of you have had this test done on routine blood tests and checkups, but you may not have known what it was for. A C-reactive protein test measures the level of C-reactive protein (CRP) in your blood. CRP is a protein made by your liver. It's sent into your bloodstream in response to inflammation. Inflammation is your body's way of protecting your tissues if you've been injured or have an infection. It can cause pain, redness, and swelling in the injured or affected area. Some autoimmune disorders and chronic diseases can also cause inflammation. There are normally low levels of C-reactive protein in your blood. High levels may be a sign of a serious infection or other disorder. Therefore, a CRP test may be used to find or monitor conditions that cause inflammation. One of those disorders is an autoimmune disorder. We will discuss autoimmune disorders later in this chapter.

# You Can Live Like This

## What This Means to Your Body, and How Fat Helps

I want to focus on how we can begin to counteract the effects of cellular inflammation. By the time you finish reading this book, I hope you will understand what a big role nutrition can play in your health and balance. This is my main goal for you. Each chapter is intended to build basic knowledge and understanding to equip you to choose a healthy balance.

Nutrition should be our priority when trying to counteract the effects of cellular inflammation. Here are some ways to do this:

- Implement an anti-inflammatory diet.
- Give our bodies well-balanced, regular daily servings of nutrient-dense foods.
- Limit pro-inflammatory foods (more about this in a bit).

## Fat Defined

Fat is very important to our health and balance, but the right *kind* of fat is crucial. Let's take some time right now to address fat.

In my opinion, fat is one of the most misunderstood components of health and balance today. I want to help clear some of the teachings and misunderstandings you may be living with. So let's delve into the subject of fat. I hope you will remember and apply these things as you begin your journey of understanding good quality fat. And I encourage you to make this a foundational piece. You will feel better for it, and this lifestyle will take on a whole new dynamic, with you feeling better than you ever knew you could!

Here is a great fact from the American Heart Association; they have something very profound to say:

> **"Dietary fats are essential to give your body energy and to support cell growth. They also help protect your organs and help keep your body warm. Fats help your body absorb some nutrients and produce important hormones, too. Your body needs fat." American Heart Association**

Please remember:

- A *balance* of good fat does not make you fat or cause heart disease.
- Deficiency in good fat leads to deficiency of the fat-soluble vitamins (A, D, E, K).
- Deficiency in good fat brings a greater risk of a variety of other ailments.

I believe it is important to have animal fats in our diets for the consumption and the absorption of fat-soluble vitamins (A, D, E, K), all of which are essential for the normal functioning of our immune system. Over the years we have moved away from consuming quality animal fats from pasture-raised animals. Such foods include butter, lard, and bacon fat, and now we find ourselves using vegetable oils. We are therefore consuming much fewer fat-soluble vitamins

# Chapter 7: Inflammation

than ever before—not to mention the almighty fat-free way of eating! We have created a phobia about fat. The problem is *not* fat, it is unhealthy fat, especially processed fats.

Fats are broken down into fatty acids in the digestive tract, and then fatty acids are broken down in our cells for energy. Fatty acids are found in the outer membrane of every cell. These different fatty acids play a role in inflammation and immunity.

Omega-6 fatty acids can be pro-inflammatory, but we *need* omega-6 fatty acids in our diets; they are essential for life! To avoid inflammation, we must strive to set a balance of the ratio between omega-6 to omega-3 fatty acids. When omega-6 fatty acids are much higher than the normal ratio, and/or the omega-3 fatty acids are much lower than the normal ratio, we are out of balance. This can be a contributor to inflammation and a large number of chronic diseases. So the solution is not to stop eating omega-6 fatty acids. The solution is to increase our consumption of omega-3 fatty acids, especially since this is where the Western diet is incredibly deficient. Some studies show that most Americans have a dietary intake of 10:1 to 25:1, mainly due to the increase in consumption of processed seed oils, grains, and the higher levels of omega-6 fatty acids that are present in the meat and dairy from grain-fed animals.

Most studies show that the ratio of the omega-6 and omega-3 fatty acids are far more important than the actual quantity of these fats, as long as you are eating enough fat to meet your daily needs. In summary, we should set a daily goal of 4 omega-6 fatty acids, to 1 omega-3 fatty acid: as in a 4:1 ratio. Some may need to keep it closer to a 1:1 – 4:1 ratio, depending on their current health status.

Fat is composed of chains of fatty acids. Fatty acids are the building blocks of fat. Amino acids are the building blocks of protein, and monosaccharides are the building blocks of carbohydrates. Fatty acids can be divided into four general categories:

**Saturated fatty acids**

These fatty acids are very stable and not easily oxidized; they are highly shelf-stable and excellent, even for high-temperature cooking, which also means eating them doesn't contribute to oxidative stress in our bodies. They are easy for the body to break apart and use for energy. The more saturated fat in a food, the better source of a fat-soluble vitamin tends to be. Examples of these fats are lard, butter, coconut oil, and palm oil. They will be solid at room temperature. let me define a few of these terms for you in case you are not familiar with them:

> *Oxidative stress* is the precursor to oxidative damage. It occurs when there is the imbalance between the production of free radicals and the body's ability to counteract their damaging effects through neutralization with antioxidants.
>
> *Antioxidants* are compounds produced in your body and found in foods. They help defend your cells from damage caused by potentially harmful molecules known as free radicals. When free radicals accumulate, they may cause a state known as oxidative stress.

## Monounsaturated fats

These fatty acids are less stable than saturated fat and are liquid at room temperature. Stability means they are less likely to go rancid, become toxic, or are more susceptible to oxidation. Monounsaturated fats require more enzymes to break them apart to be used as energy than saturated fats do. Examples of monounsaturated fats that have been associated with various health benefits are olive oil and avocado oil.

## Polyunsaturated fats

These are easily oxidized, which means they are prone to react chemically with oxygen. When they go through this reaction, the fatty acid is typically broken apart and produces oxidants called free radicals. Free radicals are unstable and can damage cells, causing illness, including various diseases and aging. As we age, we lose our ability to fight the effects of free radicals. This leads to more free radicals, more oxidative stress, and more damage to cells, which leads to degenerative processes and normal aging. So when these oxidized polyunsaturated fats are consumed, it causes oxidative damage to the body. Examples of polyunsaturated fats are flaxseed oil, corn oil, and safflower oil, which are liquid at room temperature, and are most stable when stored in a dark and cool place (light and heat can cause oxidation). Polyunsaturated fats are categorized as omega-3 and omega-6 fatty acids.

There are two essential polyunsaturated fatty acids that the body cannot make itself: Alpha-linolenic acid (ALA): omega-3 fatty acid, from which all other needed omega-3 fatty acids can be synthesized. Linoleic acid (LA), is an omega-6 fatty acid, and is where all other omega-6 fatty acids can be synthesized from. There are two main types of omega-3 fatty acids: eicosapentaenoic acid (EPA), and docosahexaenoic acid (DHA).

Omega 9 fatty acids are monounsaturated fatty acids and are beneficial in our diets too. Much less is known about how they interact with our bodies than the omega-6 and omega-3 fatty acids. Oleic acid is an omega 9-fatty acid and is found in olives, olive oil (especially cold-pressed virgin and extra virgin olive oil), avocados, avocado oil, walnuts, and macadamia nuts and has anti-inflammatory properties.

So for the sake of going further into the science, I want to discuss what *is* important regarding cellular inflammation and connected illnesses (example: autoimmune disease), where omega fatty acids are concerned. We have read that most Western diets are deficient in omega-3 fatty acids. So when our diets are deficient in omega-3 fatty acids, we have an imbalance in the ratio of omega-6 to omega-3 fatty acids. Most of this has to do with the fact that we are now being taught to consume these processed seed oils, grains, and higher levels of omega-6 fatty acids that are present in the meat and dairy from grain-fed animals.

If you are supplementing with omegas, there is no established adequate intake (AI) or dietary reference intake (DRI) in the United States for EPA and DHA omega-3s; the omega-3 fatty acid that our body can use. A growing number of experts and health professionals recommend 250 milligrams (mg) to 1,000 mg of EPA and DHA per day. I want to emphasize

# Chapter 7: Inflammation

again that I always believe our first approach should be through food, not supplementation. But many times supplementation is needed to help us get back in balance or maintain balance.

**Trans fats**

Most trans fatty acids are made through an industrial process called hydrogenation. Adding hydrogen to fat changes its texture and consistency and increases its shelf life. There is absolutely nothing healthy about this process. You will find trans fat in vegetable shortenings and some margarine, crackers, cookies, and snack foods. Intake of trans fatty acids increases blood LDL cholesterol (bad cholesterol) levels, raises the risk of coronary heart disease, and lowers your HDL (good cholesterol) levels. Your LDL should be low, and your HDL should be high to make for a healthy heart. On a side note, think for a minute about the snack foods that go into children's lunch boxes or the foods served at their school cafeteria. They are already consuming these trans fatty acids at an early age, and the negative side effects are beginning to build up in their little bodies. Remember, they are forming lifelong habits.

This leads me to canola oil. There are two sides to this story. One is a group that sees it as a healthy food, while the others avoid it at all costs. I have become one of those who take the side of avoiding this food at all costs, and this is the angle I will come from to establish my point. Supporters that believe canola oil is healthy, normally make their decision based on their belief that it is rich in omega-3 fatty acids, low in saturated fats, and is a good source of oleic acid. On a surface level, this may be true. I know how difficult it is to decipher what is healthy and what is not with so much false or confusing teaching and advertisement all around us. So I want to try to clear this confusion especially when the bottle of canola oil is labeled as being "Heart Healthy."

Most canola oil is a genetically modified product, cheap to manufacture, and many processed foods contain it. It was first created in the early 1970s as a natural oil, but over the years, with the help of Monsanto (recently bought out by Bayer), we received a genetically modified version of canola oil. Most of the crops were genetically engineered by 2009.

Canola oil works well as an industrial oil, but once it was figured out how to do genetic modification, it began being sold as an edible food product. The original oil didn't have so many negative health effects, but today the reason I see it as very harmful to our bodies is that the majority of it is genetically modified. Canola oil is normally commercially processed or is refined. I was once told by my nutrition teacher in nursing school, "You can think of hydrogenated as a liquid plastic that will block your arteries." She was right on, even in the early 1970s!

Unfortunately, I don't believe studies are showing the long-term effects of GMO canola oil on our health, but there are reports that it has caused many serious health issues over the years connected to kidneys, neurological issues, and the liver.

## You Can Live Like This

When you see "partially hydrogenated oil" on a food label, you know some amount of trans fat is present, even if the label tells you that there is zero trans fat. Trans fatty acids are hazardous byproducts of food processing and are health destroyers. At this point let me also state that canola oil has a poor omega-6 to omega-3 ratio. If you decide canola oil is not for your family, I would also suggest eliminating these hydrogenated oils or at least minimizing them: corn oil, safflower oil, soy oil, and vegetable oil.

In 2016, a bill was signed by the president of the U.S.A. amending the Agricultural Marketing Act of 1946. It caused companies to be required by law to disclose the presence of GMO ingredients through text labels, symbols, or digital links (like scannable QR codes). The only problem is that it is left up to the secretary of agriculture to decide what amounts of GMO ingredients need to be present in a food product for the GMO labeling law to be a requirement.

I will not voluntarily sign my family up to consume these. It just makes me shiver to think of the families that don't understand what is in their food. I am heartsick over the number of children who are battling serious health and even life-threatening illnesses. The numbers today are staggering. We have to educate ourselves and stop believing everything the government or these large companies are telling us. Remember, they make large sums of money off of us. I will jump off of this soapbox for now, but I can't leave it without encouraging you to be open to education and truth. There are many studies and reports available if you do your own research about food safety and health. Most likely many of you would be shocked. Do not be overwhelmed by these, or if you are not in a need to know mindset then don't even waste your energy researching. Spend your time and energy getting on a path to health, wellness and living at your optimum weight by educating yourself on healthy choices. That is the best use of your time for you and your family.

In my opinion, there are so many good fats to choose from that just a little knowledge can turn your fat intake into a health benefit.

Here are a few ideas:

- Avocado oil (cold-pressed)
- Bacon fat
- Coconut oil (typically extra-virgin, expeller pressed, but also naturally refined)
- Olive oil, organic extra-virgin
- Palm oil (which is made from palm fruit instead of the palm kernel. It should be certified sustainable and unrefined). Not to be confused with palm kernel oil.
- Pan drippings
- Poultry fat
- Red palm oil
- Organic ghee/clarified butter from grass-fed cows[4]

---

4. All ghee is clarified butter, but not all clarified butter is ghee.

## Chapter 7: Inflammation

If, for some crazy reason, you want to continue using canola oil, then make sure it is organic because then at least it's not from genetically modified plants.[5]

Since I haven't commented on grapeseed oil, I will do it here before moving on. Grapeseed oil is a high omega-6 fatty-acid oil. With that said, I would encourage you to limit it to healthy quantities and not make it your go-to oil because we have already mentioned that most of us have an overabundance of omega-6 fatty acids in our diets, and our goal is to create a healthier balance and a healthier omega-6: omega-3 ratio. If you decide to eliminate it for a time, then once you get a healthier balance you can decide when and how to reintroduce it.

So to sum this up one more way, it is not about eliminating omega-6 fatty acids, it is about balance. Balance is reducing omega-6 fatty acid, and one way is by avoiding processed vegetable oils instead of just boosting omega-3 fatty acid; with supplements. And getting omega-3 fats from whole food sources, such as wild fish, wild shellfish, and pasture-raised, grass-fed organic meats. As you seek balance, remember to focus on the *quality* of the fat first, and then the quantity of it. All omega fatty acids are not created equal. Whenever I talk about balance I am always referring to a healthy variety too; you don't want to consume the same food or the same fat regularly. Always incorporate a variety. I will go into greater detail about this in chapter 9. On a final note, let me emphasize again, whether you are consuming saturated, monounsaturated, or polyunsaturated fat, it is *always* about having a variety and balance of healthy fats in your food.

Let's talk about examples of food that are supportive of decreasing inflammation and that are high in omega-3 fatty acids. As a side note, these can also be beneficial to lowering levels of cholesterol, slowing plaque buildup in your arteries, and raising HDL (high-density lipoprotein) in your blood. Remember, HDL is considered good cholesterol. So to be balanced and healthy, you want your blood work to reveal a higher HDL count.

Examples of foods that are supportive of decreasing inflamation:

- Mackerel
- Salmon
- Herring
- Oysters
- Sardines
- Anchovies
- Caviar
- Tuna

---

5. For more information, see https://www.usda.gov/media/blog/2013/05/17/organic-101-can-gmos-be-used-organic-products

Examples of foods that contain omega-3 fatty acids that are not as high as those above:

- Walnuts
- Pastured eggs
- Meat from grass-fed animals
- Dairy products from grass-fed animals
- Hemp seeds
- Spinach
- Brussel sprouts

Examples of foods that contain omega-6 fatty acids:

- Walnuts (they are both omega-3 and omega-6)
- Tofu
- Hemp Seeds
- Sunflower seeds
- Peanut butter
- Avocado Oil
- Walnut Oil
- Eggs
- Almonds
- Pine Nuts
- Brazil Nuts

Here is an overview of some anti-inflammatory foods. Of course, those who have sensitivities and chronic health problems to any items listed below may need to eliminate or limit their intake. I will discuss eliminating foods further when I discuss Autoimmune Disease and Leaky Gut.

**Anti-inflammatory foods:**
- Fruits - the substance that gives fruits like cherries, raspberries, and blackberries their color is a type of pigment (anthocyanins) that helps fight inflammation
- Vegetables - dark leafy greens like spinach and kale, as do broccoli and cabbage.
- Whole grains (unrefined grains)
- Beans
- Nuts, olive oil, avocado oil, and avocados
- Fatty fish
- Fresh herbs and spices; examples include turmeric, curcumin, and garlic

Before moving on, I want to mention a few examples of foods that help lower LDL (low-density lipoprotein). We want our LDL blood level low. This is the bad cholesterol that, when elevated, increases our risk of heart disease and stroke.

# Chapter 7: Inflammation

- Fruits and vegetables with high fiber content
- Dark chocolate contains flavonoids and antioxidants that help lower LDL levels. Just be sure to eat in moderation, as chocolate is also high in saturated fat and sugar.
- Avocados
- Red wine (a glass)
- Almonds, walnuts, and pistachios
- Whole grains
- Plant-based fat like olive oil
- Black beans, kidneys, and lentils

When I spoke a few paragraphs ago about healthy alternative oils, it is important to also enlighten you regarding their smoke points. The smoke point means the burning point. The smoke point of an oil correlates with its level of refinement. Once you see smoke begin to come out of your pan or skillet, it means the fat has heated past its smoke point, and that fat is now beginning to break down, releasing free radicals and a chemical that gives food its acrid flavor and aroma. Now you have scorchy-tasting food. We all know that is not desirable. And it yields a fat that is now higher in free radicals, which is unhealthy.

**Smoke Points of Healthy Oils:**
- Avocado oil, cold pressed: 375°F
- Coconut oil, extra-virgin, expeller pressed, but also naturally refined: 350°F
- Olive oil, organic extra virgin, unrefined/cold pressed: 250°F - 320°F *LOW SMOKE POINT (not recommended for frying but good for salad dressings)
- Ghee/clarified butter from grass-fed: 485°F
- Beef fat/tallow, organic from grass-fed and grass-finished: 370°F - 400°F
- Pork fat/lard, organic: 370°F
- Poultry fat/schmaltz, organic: 375°F
- Palm oil: 450°F

## The Digestive System

From your mouth where the food comes in, to the opening where waste comes out, is one continuous tube. The stomach holds the food you eat until the gastrointestinal (GI) tract, called the gut, is ready to receive it. The GI tract tube includes the mouth, esophagus, stomach, small intestine, large intestine, and anus. The small intestine is where most nutrients are absorbed into the body. Nutrients are supposed to come into the small intestine, while everything else stays out. Food has to be broken down into its simplest form to cross the lining of the small intestine.

This job of breaking down food is accomplished by the combined efforts of the acid and digestive enzymes of the stomach, bile salts of the liver, and the friendly bacteria that live in the gut. To be absorbed into the body, proteins must be broken down into amino acids, fats must be broken down into fatty acids, and carbohydrates must be broken down into simple sugars (monosaccharides).

Once the food is broken down, the cells that line the gut transport nutrients from inside the gut to the rest of the body. Some vitamins and minerals are absorbed in the mouth, stomach, and large intestine. Water is absorbed primarily in the large intestine. Material not digested by the body is excreted as waste.

## Gluten

The characteristics of gluten give bread its elasticity and help it rise and keep its shape, leaving the final product with a chewy texture. Although gluten pertains only to wheat proteins, it refers to the combination of proteins naturally occurring in all grains. These include any species of wheat, barley, rye, some oat cultivars, and any cross-hybrid of these grains. Gluten comprises seventy-five to eighty-five percent of the total protein in bread wheat (also known as common wheat).

As you might imagine, the gluten our grandparents ate was an entirely different type of wheat than the super-fluffy bread that we find in grocery stores now. And today they frequently contain artificial colors, added sugar, glyphosate, and other problematic ingredients. Wheat provides some nutrients, including essential amino acids, minerals, vitamins, phytochemicals, and dietary fiber. Unfortunately, today's bread is a product of crossbreeding and genetic manipulation that began in the 1960s to create a higher-yielding, lower-cost crop. Modern wheat has also been bleached and heavily processed and thus decreases specific nutrients in wheat.

### Gluten-Free Labeling

Many have turned to foods labeled as gluten-free and think they are doing something healthy. It saddens me to inform you that gluten-free does not mean healthy or healthier. Most gluten-free products are more abundant in sugar (especially high-fructose corn syrup and table sugar), cereal grains (corn, rice, and oats), highly processed oils (canola and rapeseed oil), and commonly contain a form of soy. All in all these products contribute to the leaky gut syndrome and inflammation.

Gluten-free foods can be created at home with healthy gluten-free flours, natural sweeteners, and healthy fats, and will be an option for you as you enter Phase 2.

### Gluten-Free and Grain-Free Flours

This section is dear to my heart because gluten ended up being at the top of my list of food intolerances. I love bread, so this was disappointing at first. Then as we progressed in our journey, I learned that there were more ways than one to bake a fresh loaf of bread or other types of bread, like pumpkin or banana bread. I have enjoyed every minute of experimenting with recipes and grain free flours. I have learned that these are not all created equally. I use some alone, and others I mix one or two flours together. But the result is the same—they can all be used to make a great bread recipe!

Note: Some gluten-free flours are heavier and absorb more moisture than wheat flours, so they need a bit more liquid for the baked goods to be tender and moist.

My go-tos:

- Cassava/Yucca root
- Coconut
- Tiger Nut
- Arrowroot
- Tapioca
- Almond (Phase 3)

## Food Allergies, Sensitivities, and Intolerances

Simply stated, the difference between a food allergy and sensitivity is the body's response. When you have a food allergy, your immune system causes the reaction. If you have a food sensitivity or intolerance, the digestive system triggers the reaction. Food intolerance(s) is the one I will be referring to from this platform. The good news is that once you have eliminated all the foods you can't tolerate from your diet, you should begin to see improvement in your symptoms. Additionally, you should be able to reintroduce these foods back into your diet as early as three to six months once your gut has begun to repair and your immune system is stronger.

If you have an autoimmune disease, you will want to wait until you are in full remission. Food intolerances do not tend to be a permanent problem. Generally, this means that removing those foods from your diet for an extended period while restoring gut-barrier function will enable you to eat most of them in the future without problems. But let me go ahead and simply define all of these.

**Food Allergies:**

A food allergy is when your immune system reacts to the food as it would to a harmful invader. Your immune system kicks in, causing your cells to release a substance called immunoglobulin E (IgE) to counteract the allergen. From that point on, whenever you're exposed to that same food, your body releases histamine, which can lead to telltale allergic reactions: hives, trouble breathing, digestive problems, etc. Food allergy reactions come on quickly and have the potential to be life-threatening. The most common food allergies in the United States are to eggs, milk, peanuts, tree nuts, wheat, shellfish, and soy.

## Food Intolerances:

An intolerance to a food is an immune response other than IgE reactions (typically IgG, IgA, or IgM antibodies). When you have a severely leaky gut, proteins from anything you eat can cross the gut barrier and interact with the immune system. The more damaged your gut barrier is and the more activated your immune system is, then it is more likely for you to develop food intolerances.

While these foods don't normally irritate the gut or activate the immune system, your food intolerance will exacerbate inflammation. You may be able to figure out which food(s) you are sensitive to by eliminating the suspect(s) for two to three weeks and seeing if that makes a difference. This is simple if you consistently notice symptoms when eating a specific food. However, if there are multiple culprits, it may be a good idea to ask your health care practitioner to order a food sensitivity test and help you interpret the results. A few of the most common intolerances are dairy, eggs, legumes, cereal, grains, and nuts. Once you have eliminated all the foods you can't tolerate from your diet, you should start to see improvement. The good news is that you should be able to reintroduce these foods back into your diet as early as six months later, once your gut has healed substantially and your immune system is better regulated, although it is safest to wait until your autoimmune disease is in full remission. This will be an individual decision because each one is at a different level of illness or inflammation. Unlike food allergies, food intolerances tend to be transient. This means that by removing those foods from your diet for an extended period, along with restoring gut-barrier function, you'll be able to eat most of them in the future without problems.

## Food Sensitivities:

Food sensitivities are distinct from allergies and intolerances because they do not involve antibody production. Sensitivities may arise through various other mechanisms, including the effects of severe gut dysbiosis (production of bacterial metabolites, or from an inability to metabolize a substance). This can result from inflammation, damage to the gut, strain on the liver, or damage to other tissues.

If there is a damaged or inflamed gut, food sensitivities may develop against any food and be difficult to diagnose. There are usually no specific tests; the only way to figure it out is by eliminating it from your diet. The following are the most common food sensitivities that might be hindering your ability to have good health: FODMAP sensitivity (sometimes called fructose malabsorption), histamine intolerance, sulfite sensitivity, salicylate sensitivity, and other sensitivities specific to your autoimmune disease. These can make the healing process more challenging but not impossible.

## Leaky Gut

I'm sure you're wondering what might be going on in your body that calls for healing your gut. A common diagnosis that isn't necessarily readily recognized, even today by the

## Chapter 7: Inflammation

medical arena, is increased intestinal permeability, also known as "leaky gut syndrome." It is a digestive condition where bacteria and toxins can "leak" through the intestinal wall. This can happen when cracks or holes develop in the intestinal tract lining and, therefore, it does not work properly. This breakdown allows substances to leak into the bloodstream, leading to inflammation and contributing to some diseases, especially autoimmune disorders.

Leaky gut left unrepaired can lead to more severe health issues like inflammatory bowel disease, arthritis, eczema, psoriasis, depression, anxiety, migraine headaches, muscle pain, and chronic fatigue, to name a few, while also causing malabsorption of vital minerals and nutrients.

*I want to say this again but in different terms, because I don't want you to move beyond this point without having a clear understanding of leaky gut.*

Leaky gut takes place in your small intestine. A normal, healthy gut absorbs nutrients and keeps the nutrients inside of the gut. It separates the gut content from the rest of the body. A healthy gut uses approximately forty percent of the body's energy to do its work. On the other hand, a leaky gut reveals a breakdown of these cell walls. They become permeable, allowing these undigested foods, including bacteria, to pass into the body. When these nutrients escape the gut, it causes inflammation and possibly tissue damage. As this happens, your body's response system begins to fight.

With a leaky gut (imbalance), your body is literally fighting against itself or attacking itself, and inflammation naturally increases as this occurs—thus autoimmune symptoms. This same inflammation causes the thyroid gland to not function optimally. It can also affect all organs and systems of the body, healing, brain function, nervous system, etc. The thyroid is normally the first reactive organ. When the thyroid is not functioning at its best, it diminishes the gut's ability to repair itself. This vicious cycle reveals how important it is to restore your gut's health, support a healthy gut, and prevent a leaky gut.

I previously wrote about anti-inflammatory foods that assist in preventing or healing inflammation. Pro-inflammatory foods do the opposite. They encourage or cause inflammation. When pro-inflammatory foods are consumed regularly, they will aggravate the gut barrier. Pro-inflammatory food examples are: grain/gluten, alcohol, sugar, artificial sweeteners, high fructose corn syrup, trans fats (which are hydrogenated fats- this includes foods fried in unhealthy oils), preservatives, processed foods, especially ones high in emulsifiers, sodas, dairy (when processed or on your list of non-tolerated foods), grain-fed beef, and nonsteroidal anti-inflammatory drugs (NSAIDs), to name a few. I hope this helps bring clarity to the basics and the importance of a balanced, healthy gut.

### Autoimmune Disorders

It is mind-blowing when you learn about Autoimmune Disorders and how vast the list is.

> **According to the American Autoimmune Related Diseases Association (AARDA), there are fifty million Americans suffering from at least one autoimmune disease.**

If you are diagnosed with an autoimmune disorder, you may experience one or more of these symptoms:

- Thyroid or other organ disorders
- Pain
- Body not functioning optimally
- Autoimmune disease
- Leaky gut
- Gut dysbiosis

Approximately one out of 125 Americans have autoimmune thyroid disease, and remember this number changes every year. Your symptoms may be extreme by the time it shows in your blood work. Here are some common signs or issues you may be experiencing or have encountered, even if you are not diagnosed:

1. Bloating, gas
2. Food sensitivities
3. Thyroid conditions (such as Graves disease or Hashimoto's thyroiditis)
4. Fatigue
5. Abdominal pain
6. Joint pain
7. Headaches
8. Skin Issues like rosacea and acne
9. Digestive
10. Diarrhea
11. Weight gain

## Gut Dysbiosis

Severe gut dysbiosis may be the culprit leading to your food sensitivities and commonly precedes these reactions. Gut dysbiosis is an imbalance in your gut flora caused by too few beneficial bacteria and an overgrowth of bad bacteria, yeast, or parasites. Gut dysbiosis is said to affect thirty million Americans. It is very commonly reported as a condition in the gastrointestinal tract, particularly small intestinal bacterial overgrowth (SIBO) or small intestinal fungal overgrowth (SIFO). Both are considered a form of gut dysbiosis.

## Chapter 7: Inflammation

Gut dysbiosis is associated with the pathogenesis of both intestinal and extra-intestinal manifestation. Intestinal disorders include inflammatory bowel disease, irritable bowel syndrome (IBS), and celiac disease, while extra-intestinal manifestation (EIM) include allergies, asthma, metabolic syndrome, cardiovascular disease, and obesity.

A primary cause of poor gut health, or dysbiosis, is an unhealthy diet high in processed foods, but other practices in the modern-day world can also be contributors. Frequent use of medications such as NSAIDs like ibuprofen, multiple rounds of antibiotics, and the use of acid-blocking drugs can all contribute to an unhealthy gut environment. Chronic stress can be an additional trigger. Dysbiosis can eventually lead to other gut issues, including increased intestinal permeability or leaky gut. If ignored, gut inflammation can eventually become systemic inflammation.

**Healthy Natural Treatment for Inflamed Gut Disorders**

Since all of these gut issues are ultimately pro-inflammatory disorders, much of the content of this book can be considered a beneficial treatment to bring your body into balance and balance the microbiomes.

Here is a summary of the process:

1. **REMOVE** foods and factors that damage the gut or that you are intolerant of.
2. **REPLACE** these foods with healing foods. Include organic bone broth; it is rich in glycine, gelatin, and glutamine, which is essential for intestinal repair.
3. **REPAIR** with specific supplements as your healthcare professional suggests. These will likely include digestive enzymes or a gut repair supplementation.
4. **REBALANCE** with pre and/or probiotic supplementation (as directed by your health care advisor) and healthy bacteria-supportive foods.
5. **LISTEN TO YOUR BODY!** Now you understand better how these symptoms and changes you have been experiencing are your body just trying to get your attention.

Overall, when gut health improves, other issues or symptoms resulting from this imbalance begin to improve or disappear, such as:

- Decreased immunity
- External symptoms, including skin disorders
- Overall inflammation leading to poor health and a weak immune response
- Inability to maintain optimum weight or lose or gain weight
- Cognitive function

Gut health is such a critical foundation for vibrant health and wellbeing!

# Chapter 8

# TEID Lifestyle

Let's jump right into the nutritional aspect of how we are going to achieve this balance through the TEID Lifestyle. I know this is the chapter you have all been waiting for!

I know it took so long to get here, but there were some details I needed to cover to bring value to where you are headed. The more understanding you have, the stronger you will begin. As I mentioned earlier, the foundation is really about changing how you think. Up to this point, I have been painting a picture of a new lifestyle and mindset. New habits form as you hear something you want for yourself, then excitement comes, and you adopt it for yourself.

I created the TEID Lifestyle because I needed to make various adjustments to everything that was out there to meet my personal needs. It was simpler to identify what I felt should be included, which I soon realized went back to a healthy foundation and what can work for everyone.

In the charts following, you will notice that I have broken the nutritional part of the TEID Lifestyle into Phase 1, Phase 2, Reintroduction, and Phase 3. My definition of a phase regarding the nutritional charts in the TEID Lifestyle is a period of time, a process of change, and/or a new development. Phase 1 and Phase 2 go on for a different length of time than Phase 3. These do not last a lifetime, but long enough to learn the foundational basics of balance as you develop and make progress in your healthy lifestyle.

All of this is accomplished in your own timing. Remember, this is about you. As the processing and change take place, you will advance as your body is ready. You will move into Reintroduction and the final phase, Phase 3, when you have accomplished healing and can maintain that healing state. You now have a lifestyle that you can continue indefinitely unless you need to back up and revisit a previous phase to come back into balance. Now that you have an overview of the purpose of the various phases, let's look deeper into each of them.

In Phase 1, unless you have already been on some form of a diet regime, you should see some drastic changes to what you are currently eating. I believe with all my heart that this change is necessary. You have to turn this journey around completely, and you have some healing to do to achieve your healthy balance.

The most healing benefits will come for those of you who follow the Phase 1 lifestyle for a minimum of thirty to sixty days. Think of it as the beginning of the new you. These days will go faster than you can imagine. If you have major health issues, you may want to follow Phase 1 for sixty days or longer. You will gladly follow it if you go from dealing with constant pain to becoming pain-free or from having no energy to being more energetic. You will no longer experience the cravings you have battled for years. And when your blood sugar, blood pressure, and sleep are improving, too, you will be telling everyone about this change!

Some people will move forward more quickly into Phase 2. If you have no complaints and are here because you want to find a healthy balance, then thirty to sixty days may be the maximum time you spend in Phase 1. But this decision is up to you; listen to your body and your medical advisor. Don't be in a rush if your body is showing healing. Let your body receive the healing it needs to get on with life and not feel that you need to revisit Phase 1 because you moved on too quickly.

If you are heavier than you should be, it will be a common side effect to lose weight as you create and maintain balance. It is so beautiful how the body responds, and metabolism comes alive. *This lifestyle will allow you to achieve your optimum weight!*

At the correct time for you, you will begin Phase 3, where you maintain this balance for life. You always have the option to jump back into any phase to tighten up your weight and/or your balance. They truly go hand in hand!

If you need to gain weight but still want to find this balance, you will need to implement a few changes to accomplish this task. In Chapter 9, when I speak about vegetables, you will notice a notation in the paragraph about starchy vegetables. It says you will include more of these vegetables and may also need to increase your portion size of all foods if your goal is to gain weight. But I am guessing most people want to lose a few pounds—some more than a few—and some may just want their health back. So Phase 1 will not need any changes for the majority reading.

After you browse the phases in the TEID Lifestyle ahead, you will note that the following chapters go right into teaching about meat and vegetable choices. We have already covered fats in Chapter 7. All of this together makes for a simple healthy

# Chapter 8: TEID Lifestyle

foundation, and it also creates the knowledge within you to be able to eat anywhere and still choose a healthy balance.

*You will begin your healthy, balanced lifestyle on day one of your journey.* Take my hand as you read, and follow my lead to start your journey to your optimum weight. We are not playing around. I am focused on helping you win, and I know what it takes—no more dieting yourself into frustration, which leads to discouragement, failure, and often more weight gain. You are on a path to winning for a lifetime. I don't want you ever to have to journey this way again.

You can take charge, and I will show you how to do that. It has been said that good things in life are worth working for. You are worth working for! If you happen to find it tough in the beginning, hang on. It will get easier, and it will be so worth it. Take on a healthy mindset, one focused on you. You will appreciate this when you encounter a challenging day. You will overcome those discouraging thoughts quickly if you practice this.

Phase 1 is a very short segment of time in the scope of a lifetime. It will seem like just a blink of an eye when you look back. You will begin to transition your focus and form new habits immediately. Thank you for trusting me. Thank you for putting your blinders on. Thank you for staying focused. Now let's find the real you!

## Planning and Prepping Defines Your Win

You are going to prepare yourself ahead of time. The prepping makes all of the difference for you to be in a win-win position. Starting may seem hard, but remember your vantage point. You are reading from my point of view and many others who have succeeded. And you know now that if I can, and they can, so can you.

First, commit yourself to stay the course and to make yourself a priority—no matter what it takes. This begins the process of focusing on you. This is a brand new concept for many of you, and you will have to set some new healthy boundaries for yourself.

I will ask you to make one more commitment: For the first thirty days, I want to encourage you *not* to do some of the things people do when making similar changes. It is not uncommon to browse the Internet for more information. In this case, it will not help you, but will only confuse you. This is not like every other so-called diet. It is a lifestyle. So do not research diets and meals or recipes.

Remember earlier when I mentioned putting your blinders on? Well, just like a racehorse has blinders on its head so it does not get distracted from it's goal of the finish line, I want you to put an invisible set of blinders on yourself. *Stay focused* on where you are going! If you use this book as a guide, you will have everything you need to keep you going, learning, and winning for the next thirty days. Learn from someone who lives a successful and balanced healthy life. The fact that you're holding this book tells me that you saw something that caught your eye or the person who recommended it did. So give it a try and give it your all, and see what life-changing treasures are tucked inside!

I want you to commit to taking the time to make yourself a priority. Some might need to go back and read Chapter 5 again if it seems like a distant idea to make yourself a priority. You are beyond incredible and capable. If you don't know this about yourself, hold on—you are soon going to experience an incredible you!

## Steps of Preparation

### First Step:

Prep your kitchen, office, bedroom, car, or wherever you keep food and snacks. This is very important for *your win!* We are paving the foundational path for your success.

Go through Phase 1 and remove anything from your refrigerator and kitchen pantry (office, bedroom, and car) that is on the "Avoid" column. This is a great time to make a charitable donation to a local food pantry or to help out a family in need. If there are members of your family who will *not* be following this plan with you, then it will be extremely helpful to section off the refrigerator and pantry so each of you has an area to call your own. This act will be more valuable than you can imagine.

When you go to the refrigerator or the pantry, we will set you up to win by placing good choices (foods from the "EAT" column) in your section of the refrigerator or pantry. Let's remove all of the temptations. This will be very beneficial in the first few weeks. After that, you will be so excited about the changes you see that it would be difficult to tempt you. In the chapter with all of the testimonials, you will read about Katia's journey. She made a great decision at the beginning to have a separate refrigerator in her garage for herself while the other family members used the main refrigerator. This could be an option for you too.

This isn't a game we are playing like all of the other diets you have done before. This is the real deal, and will place you in control and in a lifestyle of success—one that can happen more quickly than you can imagine.

Here are some things to have on hand to help your journey go more smoothly:

- A scale to weigh yourself on. I like the ones that show incremental gains or losses (for instance, .2 of a pound).
- A notebook for journaling these things:
  - Daily weight
  - Menu planning

## Chapter 8: TEID Lifestyle

- Meal recording
- Grocery list (may need to include a set budget)
- Your feelings and words of encouragement to yourself

## Phase 1: TEID Lifestyle

| Food | Type | Avoid | EAT |
|---|---|---|---|
| Meat and Eggs | Protein | Grain-fed or grain-finished beef and bison, any meat with hormones, antibiotics, any meat that was fed GMO feed, fish with high mercury content, farm-raised seafood, all eggs | Organic grass-fed/grass-finished beef, organic grass-fed/grass-finished bison, organic chicken, organic turkey, all-natural pasture-raised pork, wild-caught seafood, and wild game. All meats should be antibiotic and hormone-free, includes organic bone broth |
| Fruits | Carb | Goji berries, canned fruits, dried fruits, bananas, pineapples, watermelons, mangoes, raisins, yellow plantains | All other fruit including green plantains, capers, and olives; *limit all fruits to three servings per day* |
| Vegetables | Carb | Nightshades (eggplant, tomatoes, peppers, white potatoes, etc), corn | All other vegetables |
| Grains | Carb | All | None |
| Grain-Free Flours | Carb | All | None |
| Legumes | Carb | All beans, all soy | None *See the comment on pea protein under the section below about protein shakes* |
| Dairy | Fat | All dairy, including almond milk | Unsweetened coconut milk (w/o sugar, carrageenan, or soy lecithin) |
| Nuts and Seeds | Fat | All nuts, nut butter, all seeds | Coconut |
| Beverages and Fermented Foods | | Caffeine, matcha green tea, all coffee, fermented soy products, kombucha, processed sauerkraut, kimchi, kefir | Herbal decaffeinated teas, coconut water without added sugar, unsweetened coconut milk (without sugar, soy lecithin and carageenan), sauerkraut without sugar, organic pickles (without sugar, dyes or citric acid), organic bone broth |

# Chapter 8: TEID Lifestyle

| Food | Type | Avoid | EAT |
|---|---|---|---|
| Fats | Fat | Butter, margarine, canola oil, all seed oils (including corn, soybean, and peanut oils), nut butter, ghee, grass fed butter | Avocado, avocado oil (cold pressed), coconut oil (extra virgin, expeller pressed), organic extra virgin olive oil, animal fat from pasture-raised pigs, duck, organic grass-fed/grass finished beef, bison or lamb, palm oil (sustainable and unrefined), organic ghee/clarified butter from grass-fed cows |
| Sugar and Sugar Replacements | Carb | All | None |
| Food Additives | | All | Citric acid labeled as from natural sources (lemon, orange peel...) |
| Alcohol | | All | None |
| Spices and Seasoning | | All spices derived from nightshades (chili powder, paprika, cayenne, etc.), all spices derived from seeds (anise, cumin, celery seed, coriander, dill, fennel, mustard, nutmeg, etc.) | Nutritional yeast flakes, kelp, dulse, coconut aminos, and everything not derived from nightshade or a seed, vinegars (w/o sugar) |
| NSAIDS and Other | | All NSAIDs (unless doctor prescribed), appetite suppressants, foods you have a history of severe reactions to, and foods you are allergic to | Fungi (edible) |
| Gluten-Free | | Store-bought products labeled gluten-free | None |

# You Can Live Like This

## Protein Shake, a Great Way to Begin Your Day

I encourage you to do this as you begin, even in Phase 1. Most people will agree that breakfast is the meal we give the least attention to. We grab what we can as we run out the door, jump on a conference call, or go through the nearest drive through. I believe breakfast is very important, if not the most important, meal as you begin your day. It's the foundation of the day's nutrient upload. The most common quick breakfast choices are very low in protein. A protein shake is what I use to start my day strong, and you can too. It's quite simple. I do not promote more than one shake a day because I feel your body is going to heal best with whole food.

A healthy, balanced shake that is free from unhealthy sugar substitutes and preservatives is a good way to add protein and balance to your first meal of the day. I know a good breakfast is a common problem in our busy lives. Breakfast on the run can be the most unbalanced meal many consume each day. A protein shake allows for those on the run to begin their day with a fast, delicious, solid, nutritionally dense foundation.

Think about it this way, you sleep eight hours or so (fasting all night) and you run out the door empty, so to speak. No fuel in the tank. Countless men and women go to the gym first thing in the morning. Heading to do a workout first thing in the morning is not a bad idea if you had a nutritious meal. A workout without nutrition after fasting all night is not balanced. I want to help you understand this: if you don't put nutrition into your body before working any part of your body, the only place the body can pull nutrients from is the stores that are left. This means you may end up pulling nutrients from your muscles or your bones. Or, even worse, you could increase inflammation due to lack of stores to pull from.

We all need energy to perform. Unlike fats and carbohydrates, protein cannot be stored nor can the body make protein. I can't emphasize enough how important it is to get a good breakfast with adequate protein to get you going. Don't develop a habit of omitting nutritional balance in the mornings. If you do this over and over for years, you can only imagine the imbalance and inflammation that would turn into chronic inflammation. In the long run of life, this is not a pretty picture—especially after all the hours in the gym, thinking you're strengthening your body and getting healthy.

Live preventatively with a healthy balance, and be sure to consume a variety of protein sources throughout the day, and you'll likely consume adequate protein to meet your body's needs. The TEID Lifestyle is full of balance, including protein. Because breakfast is the most common meal lacking in protein, give breakfast some consideration, for the long haul.

Currently, my favorite protein powder is pea protein. I choose a pea protein that is vegan, gluten-free, dairy-free, without chemical processing, with nothing artificial added, USA sourced, has the only ingredient listed as pea powder, and is non-GMO. Peas are not on the EWG "Dirty Dozen" list at this time; therefore, I'm not concerned with pea protein

## Chapter 8: TEID Lifestyle

powder being organic, but if it is available it is okay to choose that option. I will speak more about EWG, organic and non-organic in Chapter 9.

Peas are a great source of many nutrients, including protein, vitamin B6, iron, and some fiber, although some of the fiber is lost during the extraction of the pea protein. Pea protein is a complete protein, meaning it is a source of all nine essential amino acids, including branched-chain amino acids (BCAAs). These essential amino acids are vital for maintaining a healthy, well-functioning body.

As I mentioned earlier in the chapter on food groups, it is important to remember that protein forms a part of every cell in your body and is an important building block for your skin, muscles, bones, cartilage, and blood. Your body needs protein to build and repair tissues and produce enzymes and hormones.

Phase 1 and all phase charts show protein, fat, and carbohydrates for those who want this info.

*Even though peas are not included in Phase 1, I do allow them in Phase 1 when used in a protein shake because they are ground. The suggested use of a protein shake is one time a day, maximum. When selecting your pea protein, check the process that is used to extract it. Be certain there are no negatives such as chemical processing.

**Protein Shake Sample Recipe:**
- Pea Protein Powder (the recommended number of scoop/s for one person). I always choose the original flavor to forgo one with added flavoring or ingredients I cannot identify.
- Digestive enzymes or a digestion whole-food supplement if you are in Phase 1 and 2. You can speak with your medical or nutritional advisor on this point. And you can browse and learn how these supplements can support you in your healing process by using the link at the end of Chapter 6 under Supplements.
- ¼ cup of organic (or wild, pesticide-free) blueberries.
- ¼ of a large Hass avocado (or ½ Hass small avocado or ¼ to ⅓ Florida avocado).
- 1 cup of coconut water (that does not contain sugar or additives) or 1 cup of unsweetened coconut milk (no added sugar, no carrageenan). Even better is a half a cup of each, or ½ of one and a half cup of water. Only use coconut water and coconut milk that doesn't contain sugar, soy lecithin, or carrageenan.
- Ice cubes. The number depends on the thickness you prefer and whether you want to drink it or eat it with a spoon.

**Optional Ingredients:**
- Water

- A small handful of organic spinach or micro-greens. More on growing micro-greens in Chapter 10.
- Small pinches of herbs of your choice. I like basil and/or parsley and/or rosemary removed from the stem.
- Organic spices to give flavor and variety. For instance: cinnamon, ginger, dried orange peel, or turmeric with a dash of pepper.
- Starting in Phase 2: 1 TBSP organic cacao powder (non-alkalized).
- Starting in Phase 3: Unsweetened Almond Milk (no sugar, Soy Lecithin, or Carrageenan). Vanilla unsweetened is my favorite.

In Phase 1 or 2, I do not recommend a protein powder that contains dairy, lactose, soy, or gluten. I continue to stick with these forms of protein powder in Reintroduction and Phase 3. I never recommend a protein powder with artificial ingredients, artificial sugar, citric acid (unless it is made from citrus fruit), sugar, or preservatives. I am always looking for the protein source and the natural nutrients that it has and nothing more added or processed into it, especially chemical processing and additives.

I never recommend soy protein, due to its high concentration of phytoestrogens, of which there is much controversy and the fact that nearly all soy in the U.S. is genetically engineered. Additionally, I will mention that I have some deep-seated convictions about soy and children. I do not recommend children eating soy unless it is non-GMO.

A protein shake is good before or after a workout. And I will state again that I encourage you to keep the protein shake to one per day. I especially encourage this in Phase 1 and 2 because you are changing up habits and learning to give your body balanced whole food.

One other point on protein shakes: I encourage you to chew as you drink or eat it. Healthy digestion and nutrient absorption begin with the simple act of chewing your food. When you chew your food properly, your body releases digestive enzymes in the stomach that help to break down food so that your body can convert it into energy. Digestion is one of the most energy-consuming processes of the body, so you must help your body by doing your part. Chewing your food releases saliva and sends messages to the gastrointestinal system that food is on its way, triggering hydrochloric acid production, which helps speed up the digestive process. The lower stomach begins to relax. The stomach needs to relax before channeling food to the intestines. So a thicker shake with more ice might be a good way to introduce a shake to your morning routine and encourage you to chew as you drink.

## When to Begin Phase 2 of the TEID Lifestyle

I highly recommend that you follow TEID Phase 1 for 30-60 days. If you have an autoimmune disease, excess inflammation, major health issues, or need to lose weight; I encourage you to consider staying here for a minimum of 60 days. It is a safe place to be while setting a strong foundation. If your goal is weight loss and you only need to lose a few pounds, staying on Phase 1 is helpful for 30 days to help repair your gut. If you need to lose more, I encourage you to stay in Phase 1 until you are 20-30 pounds away from your goal weight.

Also, if you are finding that you have moved on to another phase of the TEID Lifestyle and you are struggling in any way with weight loss, experiencing an increase in pain, or simply regressing to how you felt prior to beginning this lifestyle, just jog back over to Phase 1 for a week or two. This will allow you to better identify what you are really ready for. This step will help you get a stronger grip on your choices, and also you will appreciate the next phase of the journey even more. Moving to a new phase adds new foods, and some people need more time building a stronger foundation than others. Each new phase introduces new foods and it is very important to take it slow and listen to your body.

Don't be fooled by thinking that going from Phase 1 to Phase 2 is not a big jump—it is bigger than it appears!

Why? It can be a bit of a challenge for those who love sweets and bread to begin to introduce the new natural sweeteners and the grain-free flours into this phase and maintain the balance they have learned. As you prepare your plate keep in mind you are still striving to achieve a healthy balance. Especially be mindful of your goal and listen to your body. Getting to know yourself on a deeper level during Phase 1 will help you to know what limits you are now ready to enjoy.

## Phase 2: TEID Lifestyle

| Food | Type | Avoid | EAT |
|---|---|---|---|
| **Meat and Eggs** | Protein | Grain-fed or grain-finished beef and bison, any meat with hormones or antibiotics, any meat that was fed GMO feed, fish with high mercury content, farm-raised seafood, all eggs | Organic grass-fed/grass-finished beef, organic grass-fed/grass-finished bison, organic chicken, organic turkey, all-natural pasture-raised pork, wild-caught seafood, and wild game. All meats should be antibiotic and hormone-free, includes organic bone broth |
| **Fruits** | Carb | Goji berries, canned fruits, dried fruits, bananas, pineapples, watermelons, mangoes, raisins | All other fruit, including green and yellow plantains, capers, and olives; *limit all fruits to 3 servings per day* |
| **Vegetables** | Carb | Nightshades (eggplant, tomatoes, peppers, white potatoes, etc.), corn | All other vegetables |
| **Grains** | Carb | All | None |
| **Grain-Free Flours** | Carb | All others | Cassava/yucca, tapioca, tiger nut, arrowroot, coconut; *limit to 1x per week* |
| **Legumes** | Carb | All | None *See the comment on pea protein under the section below about protein shakes |
| **Dairy** | Fat | All dairy, including almond milk | Unsweetened coconut milk (w/o sugar, carrageenan, or soy lecithin) |
| **Nuts and Seeds** | Fat | All nuts, nut butter, all seeds | Coconut |
| **Other Beverages and Fermented Foods** | | Caffeine, matcha green tea, all coffee, fermented soy products, kombucha, processed sauerkraut, kimchi, kefir | Herbal decaffeinated teas, coconut water without sugar and citric acid, unsweetened coconut milk (w/o sugar, soy lecithin, and carrageenan), sauerkraut without sugar. Coconut yogurt without sugar or sugar substitutes, organic pickles (without sugar, dyes, or citric acid), organic bone broth |

## CHAPTER 8: TEID LIFESTYLE

| Food | Type | Avoid | EAT |
|---|---|---|---|
| **Fats** | Fat | Butter, margarine, canola oil, all seed oils including corn, soybean and peanut oils, nut butter, ghee, grass-fed butter | Avocado, avocado oil (cold-pressed), coconut oil (extra virgin, expeller pressed), organic extra virgin olive oil, animal fat from pasture-raised pigs, duck, organic grass-fed/grass-finished beef, bison or lamb, palm oil (sustainable and unrefined), organic ghee/clarified butter from grass-fed cows |
| **Sugar and Replacements** | Carb | All | Coconut nectar, organic 100% pure maple syrup, date syrup, organic raw honey (local is always best) |
| **Food Additives** | | All | Citric acid labeled as from natural sources (lemon, orange peel, etc.) |
| **Alcohol** | | All | None |
| **Spices and Seasonings** | | All spices derived from nightshades (chili powder, paprika, cayenne, etc.), all spices derived from seeds (anise, cumin, celery seed, coriander, dill, fennel, mustard, nutmeg, etc.) | Nutritional yeast flakes, kelp, dulse, coconut aminos, and everything not derived from nightshade or a seed, vinegars (without sugar) |
| **NSAIDs and Other** | | All NSAIDs (unless a doctor has prescribed during this 30 days), appetite suppressants, foods you have a history of severe reactions to, the food you are allergic to | Fungi (edible), organic cacao (non-alkalized), coconut manna, can coconut cream/milk (choose a brand without sugar) |
| **Gluten-Free** | | Store-bought products labeled gluten-free | Homemade gluten-free products made with grain-free flour - *limit 1x per week* |

# You Can Live Like This

**Are You Ready to Begin Reintroduction and Phase 3 of the TEID Lifestyle?**

By now you have either achieved your goal weight and/or you are very close to it, or you have accomplished your optimum health goals. I would like to think that your pain is drastically decreased and your overall wellbeing is improved at this stage.

What if a situation arises that you have no control over? If for any reason you are forced to take a break from Phase 2 prematurely, this is a good place to land. It allows you to still eat clean and balanced. But this is not meant to encourage you to jump back and forth between the two before you accomplish your goals.

Step into Reintroduction early *only* if you have something in your life that limits you from finishing your goal and you are still trying to maintain balance. I know life can sometimes take a turn, and things happen, so if you end up in a situation where you are not at home and able to control what meal is prepared for you, you can still have a plan. In this situation, using the Reintroduction guides will set boundaries and keep you from going back to your old ways. Food reintroduction is very important. You don't want to forfeit all you have achieved. You are worth everything you have learned and applied to this point. So this is only being shared to help protect you if an unexpected circumstance arises.

For that matter, any phase can be held tightly to if a situation occurs, helping you to make the best choices possible. You are still ahead of the game by maintaining as much balance as possible. This will be more beneficial to you than you might realize.

**Reintroduction Phase of the TEID Lifestyle**

This would be used to reintroduce foods as you enter into Phase 3 and beyond. Once you have experienced poor health, indigestion, pain, or obesity and get ahead of it, it becomes more important than ever before to maintain balance. You know now that it is possible to live free of pain and maintain a good healthy lifestyle. For many, it is a better quality of life and for others, it might be life.

Being ready and able to introduce some new foods successfully can be a big boost for some. It can feel like a big accomplishment, which it is! Many have had to deal with intolerances to various foods. Maybe you didn't realize it until you removed them and began to feel better. Some have yearned for certain foods. For others, the foods you were challenged to stop eating on your journey were the foods causing some health or weight issues for you. You might have stumbled because you were addicted to them. That may sound weird to be addicted to foods; simply stated, the food had more control over you than you had over that food.

If you have been previously diagnosed with an autoimmune disease, you will want to avoid Reintroduction until your gut has made a substantial improvement. Remember, this means your body was attacking itself, which was apparent by how you were feeling.

Reintroduction is when you want to maintain the balance we learned about in Chapter 6 under the section that explains what a healthy balance looks like. If you have battled autoimmune

## CHAPTER 8: TEID LIFESTYLE

disorders for many years, don't be discouraged; you have a plan that works for you now and in time, you will most likely experience a new level of healing. Just realizing that you can be in charge and enjoy your life is a huge gift. This is great news for you!

It might be beneficial for you to use or continue to use digestive enzymes and/or some supplementation. I am not going in-depth in this book regarding these, but you can find access to these through the link in Chapter 6 where I talk about supplements. You might even need to continue some medications. Your health care advisor will help you with this. But you will certainly not require as many meds as you did before stepping into your healthy balance. Your health care advisor will make this decision too. Just remember you are not getting worse anymore—now you have hope for even greater improvement and healing. Plus, you may be able to reintroduce foods that you never thought possible to consume again, with some healing, supplementation, and medications.

I can't recommend enough that you stay with Phase 1 and Phase 2 for at least two to three months before introducing Phase 3. This is the absolute minimum, and only for those who are healthy and just trying to achieve balance or minimal weight loss. I have watched some people get impatient and move on, only to back up and start over again. *It is worth being patient and building a strong foundation before you move into Reintroduction and Phase 3.* Remember, this is not a marathon; it is a way of life that puts you in charge.

TEID allows you to fully engage in a body and lifestyle you will always feel good about, and not just for a season like when fad dieting. This is a ***lifestyle plan*** you can be successful with forever. Once you take on that mindset you have won half the battle. You will then understand it is about living in balance and not about fighting to lose weight or follow the newest diet plan. Remember, balance brings healing and weight loss, even with rare splurges of out-of-balance days or those vacations when you eat out more frequently. The TEID Lifestyle is a clean and nutritional plan for a healthy lifestyle—for life! You can follow it anywhere and anytime.

When you begin Reintroduction, I suggest that you start with foods in your list of foods that you did not tolerate. The reason for this is that if you still have an intolerance to that food, you will know you are moving forward too quickly, which reveals that your gut still needs more healing. Foods that were most likely in that list are things like nuts, seeds, eggs, alcohol, and nightshades. Of course, which foods and when you introduce them are your choice. Always gauge how you feel and how your body responds as you begin to introduce these foods. You're a step ahead of where you came from. Now you know how to listen to your body.

Here is the recommended process to reintroduce foods:

- One food at a time.
- Always keep a food journal so you know what new food was eaten in case you get symptoms that may be related.
- Write down the food, including all of the ingredients, the date, and the time you ate it.
- Write down any symptoms that may arise, no matter how minor.

- If foods in an earlier stage are not tolerated well, then do not challenge the other foods in that family at this time. (For example, if ghee caused a reaction, don't reintroduce butter, cream, fermented dairy, or other dairy products just because you didn't tolerate the ghee.) It is best to treat this result, as your body telling you it needs more healing.

It is best to wait three to seven days between each new introduction. Some people may need closer to two weeks. By now you know your body better than before.

Symptoms that will mean you need to back off and stay in Phase 2 could include:

- Previous symptoms
- New gastrointestinal symptoms
- Reduced energy or fatigue
- Food cravings, especially sugar or caffeine
- Trouble sleeping or just not feeling rested in the morning
- Headache
- Increased mucus production or postnasal drip
- Itchy eyes
- Sneezing
- Aches and pains
- Changes to skin, hair, or nails
- Mood swings, especially feeling depressed or anxious

Even having one of these symptoms can indicate that you still have one or more food sensitivity. Remember that it can take a day or two after eating food for a symptom to show up. So if you have had issues in the past, taking it slower is a better plan. If you are not well or anything abnormal has been going on—even if you have not slept well for a night or two—do not introduce a new food until you are back to normal.

Here is the process to follow for reintroducing each food:

- Select the food item.
- Be prepared to eat it two to three times in one day but then not again for a few days.
- Make your first bite small and wait up to ten or fifteen minutes before continuing with more.
- If you have any symptoms at all, do not eat anymore.
- Then eat a bigger bite and stop and see how you do.
- Wait two to three hours before trying it again.
- Now eat a normal-sized portion of the food by itself or as part of a meal.
- Do not eat that food again for three to seven days.
- Do not reintroduce another new food during that time.
- Monitor yourself for symptoms.

# Chapter 8: TEID Lifestyle

This process is even more critical for those who have had autoimmune issues or food intolerances in the past. Remember, even if it is a favorite food, it's not worth the pain or slowing down your healing, which may cause you to go backward. When in doubt, it's best to continue in the phase you were previously in for a little while longer. You may be able to tolerate a food that you have a slight sensitivity to when eaten occasionally and in smaller quantities. You might consider first reintroducing the foods you miss the most and foods that seem the least likely to cause a reaction. Of course, you should pick foods with good nutritional qualities.

Here is a recommended list you might consider following to help avoid gut issues. If you had autoimmune symptoms, then the stages of reintroduction become more of a priority:

- Egg yolks
- Legumes on Phase 3 list
- Mild-based ground seed spices
- Ancient grains
- Seeds, whole or ground
- Nuts, whole or ground
- Egg whites
- Alcohol in small quantities
- Eggplant
- Coffee
- Yogurt and kefir, raw cream
- Other dairy, including cheese; hard cheeses are generally a healthier choice
- Tomatoes
- White potatoes
- Other nightshades and nightshade spices
- Chili peppers
- Other foods you may choose to reintroduce that are not included in Phase 3

## Phase 3: the Final Phase of the TEID Lifestyle

| Food | Type | Avoid | EAT | Limit (once/week) |
|---|---|---|---|---|
| **Meat and Eggs** | Protein | Grain-fed or grain-finished beef and bison, any meat with hormones or antibiotics, any meat that was fed GMO feed, farm-raised seafood | Organic grass-fed/grass-finished beef, organic grass-fed/grass-finished bison, organic chicken, organic turkey, all-natural pasture-raised pork, wild-caught seafood, and wild game. All meats should be antibiotic and hormone-free, includes organic bone broth, organic eggs (with certified humane seal) | Fish with high mercury content |
| **Fruits** | Carb | | All other fruit, including capers and olives | Can fruits in natural juice |
| **Vegetables** | Carb | Corn (with GMO) | All other vegetables, including non-GMO corn | |
| **Grains** | Carb | All grains containing gluten | Gluten-free only, including gluten-free ancient grains | |
| **Grain-Free Flours** | Carb | | Cassava/yucca, tapioca, tiger nut, arrowroot, almond, plantain, taro, yam, coconut | If still desiring to lose weight |
| **Legumes** | Carb | All soy, all peanuts, all legumes with a non-edible pod | Green beans, peas, snow peas, sugar snap peas, and scarlet runner beans, all legumes with an edible pod | |
| **Dairy** | Fat | All other dairy | Coconut milk, almond milk, coconut water (w/o sugar, sugar substitutes, carrageenan, or soy lecithin). Organic ghee/clarified butter. Coconut or almond yogurt without sugar substitutes. Organic yogurt, cheese, organic raw cream, and organic whole milk, all made from grass-fed/grass-finished cows, sheep, or goats. Herbal decaffeinated teas, homemade sauerkraut without sugar | |
| **Nuts and Seeds** | Fat | Peanuts | All forms of coconut, whole nuts, or ground nuts, as in nut butter, seeds | |
| **Beverages and Fermented Foods** | | Fermented soy products | Sauerkraut, kefir, caffeine, teas, coffees, kombucha, kimchi, pickles, organic bone broth | |

## CHAPTER 8: TEID LIFESTYLE

| Food | Type | Avoid | EAT | Limit (once/week) |
|---|---|---|---|---|
| Fats | Fat | Conventional butter, margarine, and liquid margarine, processed and refined seed oils (including corn, soybean, and peanut oils) | Avocado, avocado oil (cold-pressed), coconut oil (extra virgin, expeller pressed), organic extra virgin olive oil, animal fat from pasture-raised pigs, duck, grass-fed/grass-finished beef, bison or lamb, organic ghee/clarified butter from grass-fed cows, butter made from 100% grass-fed cows or bison, and nut butters | Seed and nut oils (sesame, macadamia, walnuts, etc.) |
| Sugar and Sugar Replacements | Carb | All | Coconut nectar, organic 100% pure maple syrup, date syrup, blackstrap molasses (unsulphured), organic raw honey (local is always best), coconut palm sugar, Xylitol | |
| Food Additives | | Do your best to avoid or limit canned items, preservatives, and citric acid | Citric acid labeled as from natural sources (lemon, orange peel, etc.) | |
| Alcohol | | | Wine, grain-free/gluten-free based spirits, mead, and beer | Grain-based spirits, beer |
| Spices and Seasoning | | | All spices, including coconut aminos, nutritional yeast flakes, kelp, dulse, vinegars, and mustard | |
| Other | | Foods you have a history of severe reactions to, the food you are allergic to, all appetite suppressants | Fungi (edible), coconut manna/butter, canned coconut cream/milk without added sugar. Organic cacao, dark chocolate, and cocoa (all non alkalized) | |
| Gluten-Free | | Store-bought and bakery products labeled gluten-free | Homemade gluten-free products made with grain-free flour, or gluten-free ancient grains | |

# Chapter 9

# NUTRITIONAL BALANCE DEFINED

This chapter will get down to the nitty-gritty of the foods on the "EAT" and "Avoid" lists and explain them more in-depth. Since the previous chapters talked about balance, it's now time to see a healthy balance in your foods. I want to also comment regarding packaged foods labeled "organic." This is where label reading, especially the ingredient portion of the label, becomes very important. So many of these items you might find listed are not actually clean foods. They still contain things you may not find on the different phases or even want to incorporate back into your lifestyle because you have become aware of better choices.

### Organic versus Non-Organic

EWG (Environmental Working Group) is an American activist group specializing in research and advocacy in agricultural subsidies, toxic chemicals, drinking water pollutants, and corporate accountability. They are a nonprofit organization that I use for my guidelines while deciding whether the produce I purchase will be organic or non-organic.

I encourage you to check out their website for yourself and carry the Dirty Dozen and Clean 15 lists with you when shopping until you have it memorized. *These lists are updated annually*, so keep track whenever the list is updated. I feel their research is accurate and current, therefore, I trust that the Clean 15 does not need to be organic. On the other hand, *I do not buy any Dirty Dozen produce without it being organic—period!* I make adjustments and change up a recipe as needed.

The 2022 Dirty Dozen List:

- Strawberries
- Spinach
- Kale, collard, and mustard greens
- Nectarines

- Apples
- Grapes
- Bell and hot peppers
- Cherries
- Peaches
- Pears
- Celery
- Tomatoes

And the 2022 Clean 15 List:

- Avocados
- Sweet corn
- Pineapple
- Onions
- Papaya
- Sweet peas (Frozen)
- Asparagus
- Honeydew melon
- Kiwi
- Cabbage
- Mushrooms
- Cantaloupe
- Mangoes
- Watermelon
- Sweet potatoes[6]

## GMO versus Non-GMO

GMO stands for "genetically modified organism." Non-GMO refers to a product produced without genetic engineering and its ingredients are not derived from GMOs. These crops have been bred using traditional crossbreeding methods found in nature.

Most GMOs have been engineered to withstand the direct application of herbicide and/or insecticide. However, new techniques are now being used to artificially develop other traits in plants, including resistance to browning in potatoes. Some crops have genetically modified versions that are widely commercially produced. Examples are corn, soy, cotton, canola, alfalfa, papaya, potato, sugar beet and zucchini. Many GMO crops are refined and turned into processed ingredients such as corn starch, corn syrup, canola oil, sugar, molasses, soy lecithin, citric acid, flavorings, vitamins, and anything that says "vegetable" but is not specific may be included.

---

6. See the EWG website for more information: https://www.ewg.org.

# CHAPTER 9: NUTRITIONAL BALANCE DEFINED

I want to conclude this topic by adding that GMOs are prohibited in organic products. For example; the organic farmer cannot plant GMO seeds, an organic cow cannot eat food produced with GMO seed, and an organic soup producer can't use any GMO ingredients. It is important to consider that they can add unhealthy oils, fats, etc. Therefore, it's important to read and have an understanding of the nutrition facts label on the food we buy. I will cover this more in depth at the end of this chapter.

## Meat

Let me begin by stating that I support the consumption of meat—healthy meat. So as I describe meat in this section, I will include some specific details for you to pay close attention to.

First, I want to cover a little science on a few details you will see repeated in this chapter. When you read the same thing over and over, know that it is important; that's how I intend the repetition to come across in this section. It separates the clean, healthy meats from the others not listed.

Grass-fed meat comes from animals that feed from grass. Examples we will see mentioned: cattle, bison, and sheep, etc. The animals should roam freely, usually within the confines of a fenced pasture, but they are not restricted in their normal movement or activities. They are usually not given antibiotics or hormones. When purchasing the finished meat, the packaging should state that it is "organic" and "100% grass-fed" and/or "grass-finished." If it doesn't state this, most likely the meat is grain-finished and is not considered 100% grass-fed meat. Grain completely changes what you are consuming. The reason I included organic is that the ground on which they are raised is to be clean and free of pesticides. Most importantly, grass-fed can be organic, but the opposite is not always true; organic does not mean grass-fed. My second choice is grass-fed/grass-finished if I can't find organic in my stores or locally grown.

Pasture-raised meat comes from animals that feed on plants and grass. Some examples you see here are pig and chicken. This means they are raised on a pasture and allowed to roam freely. Their diets will be supplemented with grains, seeds, soy, household scraps, or leftovers from a harvested crop. The supplemental feedings may or may not be organic and non-GMO. I encourage you to purchase organic and non-GMO when available. These animals usually won't do well without some supplementation, and are usually not given hormones or antibiotics.

So often I hear the terms *grass-fed* and *pasture-raised* interchanged, but they don't mean the same thing. *Grass-fed* means pasture-raised; but *pasture-raised* doesn't mean grass-fed, as you read above where pasture-raised animals are usually supplemented with grains, etc. Keep in mind that a grass-fed animal like a cow can be finished on grass or grain. If it is finished on grain, it is no longer considered grass-fed but would now only be regarded as pasture-raised.

## YOU CAN LIVE LIKE THIS

So the bottom line is to look for grass-fed and grass-finished beef, bison, or lamb and look for pasture-raised pork, chicken, and turkey. Additionally, these two types of animals (grass-fed and pasture-raised) are better choices for you to consume because they are treated better, have more vitamins and minerals, and the animals are happier and healthier. Grass-fed meat has been known to have far less E. coli contamination compared to conventional meat, mostly because animals raised on the pasture generally have healthy intestines when compared with animals raised in a feedlot that are grain-fed. The grass-fed animal isn't going to be treated with antibiotics and hormones that are routinely used in conventional feedlots, for obvious reasons.

When it comes to supporting the environment, there is a huge difference between supporting smaller farms versus the industrial farms that are leaching fertilizers and pesticides into our waterways. Grass-fed and pasture-raised meat tends to be more nutritionally dense, which means more vitamins (especially vitamin D), minerals, and a more balanced omega-6 to omega-3 fatty acid ratio. The fats of grass-fed and pasture-raised animals are much healthier. This meat may contain approximately four times more omega-3 fatty acids, which is going to lend to a better balance for you and your heart health. Also, grass-fed meat is less subject to oxidation, meaning it will have more color, longer storage life, and a better flavor.

I will make one last comment about grass-fed and grass-finished meat. If a cow that has been raised on the grass its entire life is finished off with even a few weeks of grain feeding to change up the flavor, increase the marbling in the meat, or fatten it up, the omega-6 to omega-3 ratios are changed from a desirable ratio with grass-fed to conventional grain-fed meat consistency. This is not your healthiest option. This change undermines the health benefits of the meat from a grass-fed and grass-finished animal. For this reason, again, I like to see the words *grass-fed* and/or *grass-finished* on the packages of meat I purchase.

Whenever you have the opportunity to visit the farm you get meat from or even choose your meat from, it is always an advantage for you. You can see firsthand the care and handling of the animals, the feeding process, and whether they truly are out roaming in a pasture or not. In addition to the obvious things mentioned above, if you're visiting a farm to inquire about pasture-raised animals (pig, boar, and birds) I would encourage you to ask the farmer what the animal's diet is being supplemented with. This allows you to take into consideration things you may know you do not tolerate, to find out if it is being fed non-GMO feed, and understand the nutritional qualities of the meat you can expect to get from that animal.

Here is a great link to help you find a farm in your area: www.eatwild.com.

I know that many programs do not support beef being eaten regularly. I believe meat is a healthy form of protein. The problem, especially with beef, is that grain-fed fat is not a healthy option and is an agent to cause or increase heart disease. The benefit of grass-fed beef is that it is a healthy fat that your body knows how to use and will not cause the same heart health issues that grain-fed meat causes.

# Chapter 9: Nutritional Balance Defined

I meet people every day who have walked away from eating meat. I get this. Their bodies didn't feel good because the grain-fed meat they were consuming did not strengthen their immune system but instead, caused chronic inflammation. Many times when these same people have seen or read about the feed lots and the harsh environments that many animals are raised in today, they cannot bear to support the industry or even put one bite of that kind of meat into their mouth. I completely understand!

This next bit of info is, for me, the most important point I am going to make about meat. Poultry, in general, has the worst omega-6 to omega-3 fatty acid ratio of all meat sources to choose from. And chicken is higher in bacteria. Even free-range poultry has this poor omega ratio. This is not to say that you shouldn't eat poultry; it has nutritional value. What it does mean is that poultry should not be the main source of your daily protein. Remember, it's all about balance and variety. If you do consume poultry regularly, then be sure to consume plenty of healthy seafood to balance your omega-6 to omega-3 fatty acids.

One more key point on chicken: I always purchase organic chicken when purchasing from the grocery store and I can't go to the farm to buy pasture-raised birds, seeing what the bird was fed and how it is raised. I do not want to eat GMO foods, and the only way I can be certain of this is by choosing organic options. It is important to note that organic chicken is not washed in the chemicals that non-organic chicken is washed in.

The USDA sets standards of what organic includes, and I encourage you to read up and educate yourself.[7] Take ownership of how your body is fed and taken care of. As I mentioned above, living preventively is much simpler than fixing the issue that arises from neglect.

Unfortunately, almost all weight-loss diets and programs promote a high, if not a complete, diet of chicken. This robs people of the essential nutrients found in red meat and fish and causes their omega-6 to omega-3 fatty acid ratio to be way out of balance. Today's conventionally raised chicken ratio is even higher and more out of balance than in years past. Of course, what their diet is supplemented with plays a major role. Keep in mind that most companies are going to use the least expensive avenue of supplementation than would be used with pasture-raised chickens.

Your body is looking for variety. If you want to wake up your metabolism, lose weight, or just want to get balanced, then give your body a healthy balance of nutrients to work with. When eating chicken, and this is probably the only time I am going to say this, the leaner cuts of chicken are the better cuts because they are lower in omega-6 fatty acids. So when you choose chicken, pick the breasts. The skin is also going to add to the omega-6 fatty acids, so if you are striving for balance, do not eat chicken all the time and don't always consume all or any of the skin. Again, I know you might be tired of hearing this, but it is about balance and variety. Some of you reading this will say, "But the skin is the best part!" Yes, I know;

---

7. Read more about this here. https://www.usda.gov/media/blog/2013/05/17/organic-101-can-gmos-be-used-organic-products

my husband and brother-in-law will agree with you. If you eat a balanced diet regularly, then this isn't as much of a concern as it might be for the average guy or gal—*on rare occasions*.

Now for everyone's favorite: bacon. The best bacon to consume will be naturally cured or uncured from pasture-raised animals. Bacon can be labeled as cured or uncured. Uncured bacon is bacon that hasn't been cured with sodium nitrites. This bacon will normally be cured with a form of celery, which contains natural nitrites, along with sea salt and other flavorings like parsley and beet extracts. Uncured bacon has to be labeled "Uncured bacon. No nitrates or nitrites added." However, that doesn't mean it doesn't have nitrites from naturally occurring sources.

Have you ever wondered why nitrites are added to food in the first place? Along with making bacon pink, nitrites maintain bacon's flavor, prevent strong odors, and delays the growth of the bacteria that cause botulism. Nitrites also occur naturally in some foods, including many vegetables. Vegetables do not carry the risks that nitrites do when added to meats in curing, because they tend to contain a lot of vitamin C. They also contain many other healthy vitamins, minerals, and antioxidants. In the highly acidic environment of your stomach, nitrites can be converted to nitrosamines, a deadly carcinogen. However, vitamin C appears to prevent this conversion. Since the vegetables that contain nitrites also have high levels of vitamin C, eating them sidesteps the risks involved in eating lots of high-nitrite foods that don't contain vitamin C.

Wild fish are a great way to balance out the omega-6 in your diet, especially when you consume salmon, which is high in DHA and EPA omega-3 fatty acids. Always check the ingredients to make certain that no food dyes are added. I also prefer no preservatives when I buy seafood, especially when frozen. If you don't like seafood, give it another try. If you are allergic and can't eat it, then be sure to get your DHA and EPA from good sources. The best sources of DHA and EPA are wild-caught salmon (fresh or canned), sardines, albacore tuna, trout, or mackerel.

I know there is some controversy about mercury content in certain fish, so let's address it. Methylmercury, an organic form of mercury, is the predominant form of mercury in fish. Fish at the lower end of the food chain tend to have lower levels of mercury, and fish that eat other fish tend to have higher concentrations. Now that I understand this better, it seems that the mercury in most seafood isn't as much of an issue as I thought because these foods generally contain a high selenium content. Selenium is an essential mineral that supports the immune system, fertility, and cognitive function. Mercury and selenium are found in many foods we eat other than fish. Methylmercury irreversibly binds to selenium. Most ocean fish that we eat contain much more selenium than methylmercury. This is good news because selenium-bound methylmercury is not efficiently absorbed by our bodies.

The fish I would not choose often are whale, shark, swordfish, marlin, king mackerel, sailfish, tilefish, and orange roughy, only because it is believed that their selenium levels have not been measured.

# Chapter 9: Nutritional Balance Defined

The bottom line is that it's always about balance and variety. Regardless of which fish are higher in mercury and lower in selenium, you don't ever want to eat the same fish every day. We are looking for balance and a variety of nutrients. The Environmental Protection Agency undertakes surveys of freshwater and saltwater fish. I encourage those of you that want to know more, to follow their updates.

Farm-raised versus wild seafood is another controversial subject. I do not eat farm-raised fish unless I am dining out and that is my only option. I only prefer farm-raised seafood on very rare occasions. I do not desire the GMO of farm-raised fish. But let me make the point that if that is all you have access to, then this may be an area of compromise for you. Again, we are talking about balance, and depending on your diet it may be important to consume whatever seafood you have access to for omega-3 fatty acid intake. I like to consume fish a few times a week. My favorite is wild salmon with a sprinkle of coconut aminos. I will show this in the Meal Sample section.

## Vegetables, Fiber, and Fruit

Vegetables and fruits are as important in your diet as meats and fats. Or said another way, carbohydrates are just as important in your diet as protein and fat. They are loaded with nutrients and contain essential sources of antioxidants, vitamins, minerals, and fiber. These foods give us energy, keep our bowels functioning properly (especially the fibrous produce), and help our brains work better. These are just a few of the benefits of these tasty foods.

The fiber content of produce is very important and helps to regulate hunger hormones and helps to bring gut micro-flora to a normal balance. You will notice in the TEID Lifestyle that I suggest eliminating certain foods in Phase 1 and Phase 2, and then in Reintroduction and Phase 3, listening to your body to help you determine how well your body tolerates these food items as you gradually reintroduce them. I suggest you reintroduce each one, one food item at a time to see how you do. Some foods will likely need further limitation or elimination. For example, my system struggled with processing legumes. As you have seen on the TEID Lifestyle, I suggest eliminating or limiting foods like legumes, nightshades, corn, soy, and white potatoes. I continue to limit some of these food items in my diet simply because my body feels better with smaller amounts or total elimination; and how I feel matters to me. I am thankful that I have learned to listen to my body, and you will be too!

If you experiment with many types of veggies and fruits you will be amazed at the limitlessness of the delicious variety of produce that is available, especially when following seasonal options. For most of us, we only eat a fragment of what is available and tend to eat the same foods regularly. Adding a wide variety of produce and mixing it up regularly is such an asset to your body. Just think of the plethora of healthy vitamins and nutrients you will be eating. It's so much more valuable to your body than trying to substitute nutritional lack with a man-made supplement. In a few pages when I talk about micro-greens, you will be amazed at the dense nutrient value you can easily have within reach, right at home.

## You Can Live Like This

As I make these next points, I know several things will go against the grain of what you have been taught. Many of you have come to believe that vegetables are full of carbohydrates and are bad for you, or that there are only special times to eat them, like when you are trying to load up on energy for the long haul. This is one of the reasons I don't focus totally on protein, fat, and carbohydrate balance in each meal. I want you to learn to look for balance and variety and color no matter where you are and what you have to pick from.

As I have stated in the previous paragraph, Carbohydrates play a significant role in your healthy balance. I will not tell you to eliminate these from your diet as others may because they are essential to your body. And just like all other food types, it is about finding daily balance. When you look at each produce item individually, many of you will be surprised to find what a variety of nutrients are found in each of them.

When cooking vegetables, use as little water as possible. Steaming gives a healthier result than boiling because when boiled, the nutrients end up in the water, which is usually discarded. The crunchier vegetables are when you remove them from the stovetop, the more nutrients are still left inside of them.

Here is a breakdown below using the points I want you to remember.

**Fiber**

This is a form of carbohydrate known as *roughage* or *bulk*.

Fiber plays an important role:

- Helps regulate digestion
- Helps maintain bowel health, normalize bowel movements, and prevents constipation
- Increases absorption of magnesium
- Helps control systemic inflammation
- Contributes to happy and normal gut micro-flora
- Helps control blood sugar
- Helps lower cholesterol
- Aids in achieving a healthy weight
- Reduces risk of:
    - Obesity
    - Cancer, especially colon cancer
    - Heart disease, stroke, and high cholesterol
    - Diabetes

CAUTION about adding too much fiber, too quickly; it can promote:

- Intestinal gas
- Abdominal bloating and cramping

# Chapter 9: Nutritional Balance Defined

It's important to note that you should consider increasing the fiber in your diet gradually over a few weeks. This allows the natural bacteria in your digestive system to adjust to the change in your diet. These symptoms occur because bacteria within the colon produce gas as a by-product of their digestion of fiber. There are different sources of fiber, and the type of fiber varies from source to source. The better-digested fiber produces more gas. *It's all about finding your healthy balance.* Fiber happens to be something that many people only have in scant amounts in their diet every day. This is due to all of the processed foods eaten on the run and the lack of natural fresh produce consumed daily.

**Types of Fiber:**

Your body needs two types of fiber: soluble and insoluble. Both come from plants and are forms of carbohydrates. But unlike other carbohydrates, fiber can't be broken down and absorbed by your digestive system. Instead, as it moves through your body, it slows digestion and makes your stools softer and easier to pass. Another benefit of this slowing of digestion is that it will help decrease hunger pangs and make you feel full longer.

Most foods contain both soluble and insoluble fiber but are usually richer in one type than the other. The easiest way to tell them apart is that soluble fiber absorbs water, turning it into a gel-like mush, like when water is added to oatmeal. Examples of foods with this fiber are oats, peas, beans, apples, citrus fruits, carrots, and barley. Insoluble fiber doesn't absorb water; think of adding water to celery. Insoluble fiber promotes the movement of material through your digestive system and increases stool bulk, so it can be of benefit to those who struggle with constipation or irregular stools. Soluble carbohydrates, proteins, and fats are digested in the stomach and small intestines with the help of enzymes while insoluble carbohydrates or fiber portion is digested through bacterial fermentation in the large intestine.

Each body is very individual, just like each of our gut bacteria. So it's important to experiment with various fibers and listen to your body to see which ones it tolerates best initially, and continue from there.

Here are examples of some fibrous produce options:

- Apples (include the skin)
- Oranges
- Strawberries
- Raspberries
- Exotic fruits
- Dark colored vegetables; the darker the veggie the higher the fiber
    - Carrots
    - Beets
    - Broccoli

- Collard greens
- Swiss chard
- Artichoke
- Sweet Potato (include the skin)

**Green Leafy Vegetables**

These are carbohydrates with *no limit* in the TEID Lifestyle. They are great sources of iron, calcium, potassium, magnesium, phosphorus, manganese, and even some omega-3 fatty acids. These vegetables support the immune system. It is important to note that the calcium in some leafy greens, such as kale, is extremely absorbable, even better than the calcium found in milk! Feel free to add these vegetables in a variety of courses to *every meal*, if you so desire!

- Beet greens
- Bok choy
- Broccoli rabe
- Brussel sprouts
- Cabbage
- Carrot tops
- Celery
- Dandelion greens
- Endive
- Kale
- Lettuce
- Mustard and collard greens
- Napa cabbage
- Radicchio
- Spinach
- Sweet potato greens
- Swiss chard
- Turnip greens
- Watercress

**Non-Starchy Veggies:**

These are another form of carbohydrates. They are rich in vitamins, minerals, and antioxidants.

Typically these are the stems, flowers, or flower buds of various plants rather than the leaves.

Most non-starchy vegetables fall into the low glycemic index category.

# Chapter 9: Nutritional Balance Defined

Examples of non-starchy vegetables are:

- Artichoke
- Asparagus
- Broccoli
- Caper
- Cardoon (also called the artichoke thistle or globe artichoke)
- Cauliflower
- Celery
- Fennel
- Rhubarb (stems)
- Squash blossoms
- Tomatoes
- Zucchini

**Roots, Tubers, and Bulb Vegetables**

These can be starchy or non-starchy.

Examples of these veggies include:

- Arrowroot
- Bamboo shoot
- Beets
- Carrot
- Cassava/yuca
- Ginger
- Horseradish
- Jicama
- Jerusalem artichoke/sunchoke (great prebiotic)
- Parsnip
- Radish
- Rutabaga
- Sweet potato, white sweet potato
- Taro
- Turnip
- Yam
- Water Chestnut

## Vegetables from the Onion Family:

These are particularly aromatic and flavorful and create a tasty dish, but they also contain many nutrients, such as antioxidants, calcium, iron, manganese, selenium, many B vitamins, and vitamin C.

Examples of these veggies are:

- Chives
- Garlic
- Leek
- Onion
- Shallot

## Starchy Vegetables:

It is important to note that not all carbohydrates are created equal. Starchy vegetables have a higher sugar content than other vegetables. I recommend that you **do not** commonly combine starchy vegetables in the same meal with fruit, especially the higher glycemic fruits. This is especially important if you have blood sugar issues, as in diabetes. When you are striving to maintain a balanced blood sugar level or to lose weight, watch your starchy vegetable intake and your high glycemic fruit intake. All of us should be mindful to keep a balance. These can cause you to get hungry sooner than normal, have cravings, and they will affect or slow your weight loss.

- Beets
- Beans
- Carrots
- Parsnip
- Plantain
- Pumpkin
- Yams, sweet potato
- Taro
- Squash:
    - Acorn
    - Buttercup
    - Butternut
    - Hubbard
    - Spaghetti

# Chapter 9: Nutritional Balance Defined

**Sea Vegetables:**

These are a great source of iodine and also contain calcium, magnesium, potassium, sodium, iron, chromium, and copper. They have especially high concentrations of trace minerals, vitamins, and even omega-3 fatty acids, which is unusual for plants.

Some examples of sea vegetables include:

- Dulse
- Sea kale
- Sea lettuce
- Kelp

**Nightshade Vegetables:**

The flowers, fruit, and foliage of the nightshade family contain steroidal drugs. There may be some health benefits, but it is also known to be a potent irritant both externally and internally. The vast majority of people will have no issues with nightshades, but they can be a problem for those struggling with inflammation, digestive sensitivity, gut permeability, or an autoimmune disease. Since the TEID Lifestyle removes foods that may increase inflammation or sensitivities, nightshades are eliminated until Reintroduction. For those who know they are only slightly sensitive, it might be enough just to reduce or limit nightshades in their diet.

Here are some ways to reduce some of the levels of the problematic chemicals from the food list below:

- Peel all potatoes (does not include sweet potatoes)
- Avoid green tomatoes and unripe nightshades
- Cook nightshade vegetables when you do eat them

In summary, in the TEID Lifestyle, we are concerned with inflammation, bringing about healing to this inflammatory response, and finding balance so that your body can function like it was created to do. Of course, if you are already dealing with an autoimmune disease or inflammatory disorder, this becomes more of a focus. Therefore, I do not recommend nightshades until you begin Reintroduction and Phase 3. Then be mindful to listen to your body and sense how it is tolerating these foods. My main concern is to address the potential to increase inflammation that nightshades have. Therefore, avoid them during Phase 1 and 2. This helps encourage healing in the areas of need. Certain nightshade vegetables can be excellent sources of nutrients, including vitamins, protein, and fiber, and not be an issue when you are not focused on healing inflammation.

Nightshade examples:

- Ashwagandha
- Bell peppers (sweet peppers)
- Bush tomatoes

- Eggplant
- Goji berries
- Hot peppers
- Paprika
- Pimentos
- Potatoes (does not include sweet potatoes)
- Tomatoes

If a person wishes to eliminate nightshades from the diet, they can replace them with other non-nightshade vegetables, such as:

- Sweet potatoes/yams
- Cauliflower
- Mushrooms

## Cruciferous Vegetables:

If you are currently dealing with an autoimmune disorder or low thyroid function, some experts advise that you should avoid cruciferous vegetables; which are many of the most antioxidant, vitamin, and mineral-rich vegetables available. Their reasoning comes from the goitrogenic properties these cruciferous vegetables have. Goitrogens are compounds that suppress the function of the thyroid gland by interfering with iodine uptake. Iodine is a necessary component of thyroid hormones. Thyroid hormones have essential roles in metabolism and even in regulating the immune system, so supporting optimal thyroid function is important for healing and general health. After much research, I feel eliminating these vegetables is not well justified. You may want to limit them or do an elimination test for some time.

They include:

- Arugula
- Bokchoy
- Broccoli
- Brussels Sprouts
- Cabbage
- Cauliflower
- Collard, mustard, and turnip greens
- Watercress

## Calcium-Rich Vegetables:

During Phase 1 and 2, this is more important to pay attention to because you are avoiding dairy.

# Chapter 9: Nutritional Balance Defined

- Canned salmon or sardines with bones
- Broccoli rabe
- Kale
- Broccoli
- Sweet potato
- Okra
- Mustard greens
- Collard greens
- Blackberries
- Dark leafy greens
- Butternut squash
- Edamame, non-GMO
- Dried figs

**Fruit:**

The key point I want to make about fruit is that not all fruits are created equal when it comes to eating fruit as a snack or in combination with other fruits and vegetables in a meal. Fruits will most likely fit into one of two categories: high or low glycemic, meaning how much impact a fruit will have on your blood sugar level. If you are diabetic, this matters immensely. If you are trying to get to your optimum weight and balance your body's metabolism, this matters. And if you are seeking to improve your recent blood work, ex: A1c this matters. The A1c test is a blood test that provides information about your average blood glucose levels, also called blood sugar, over the past ninety days.

Examples of **low** glycemic fruits:

- Grapefruit
- Apples
- Pears
- Oranges
- Plums
- Strawberries
- Peaches
- Blueberries
- Nectarines

Examples of **high** glycemic fruits:

- Pineapple
- Cherries
- Mango

# You Can Live Like This

- Papaya
- Grapes
- Watermelon
- Cantaloupe
- Many canned fruits (read the label to be sure there is no added sugar)
- Dried fruits such as raisins, dates, and dried cranberries (read the label; many dried fruits have oils and/or sugars added to them)

Please note that usually the riper the fruit, the more its glycemic index will increase; as in a greenish banana versus a yellowish-brown banana.

## Blood Sugar Balance

The highs and lows of blood sugar affect many parts of the body. As you seek balance, maintaining a balanced blood sugar level is important. This is one of the reasons you will begin by eating every three hours alternating a meal with a snack. Eating regularly not only helps to rev up your metabolism, introduce nutritional balance without increasing inflammation in your body, but it also helps to maintain a healthy blood sugar. I cautioned above about combinations of high glycemic vegetables and high glycemic fruits (examples shown above under the section about fruit), being consumed in the same meal. So to help you understand the value of a balanced blood sugar, I provide a few examples of what can be affected during a blood sugar imbalance:

- Stimulation of hunger hormones
- Cravings increase
- Store fat instead of burning it
- Burn muscle
- Emotional imbalance
- Lack of mental clarity

## Eating Seasonally

Eating seasonally refers to the times of the year when the harvest or the flavor of a given type of food is at its peak. Normally foods in season will be at a better price. There are many benefits to eating seasonally. When fruits and vegetables are picked for consumption where they have been naturally ripened on the vine or the tree and harvested at the right time, they will have much more flavor and nutritional value. It is also important to note that the longer produce sits on the shelves, the more nutrients and antioxidants they seem to lose. Since seasonal fruits and vegetables retain more nutrients than their counterparts this makes them the better choice for your health. Eating seasonally also supports local farmers who choose

# Chapter 9: Nutritional Balance Defined

to farm sustainably. For seasonal produce, you can use farmer's markets or local farms to purchase your produce rather than the grocery store.

Variety can keep your diet from getting boring and out of balance while giving your body a variety of healthy nutrients that help maintain a healthy balance. Unfortunately, today we have various produce available year-round because of greenhouse production. This is not all bad, I want to point out that some are ripening the fruit with the use of gas. Need I say anymore? I, for one, do not enjoy produce that tastes like a cotton ball and simply has no flavor.

I realize that for many, it is difficult to know what is seasonal because some produce is available all year long. When I was growing up and while I was raising my children, we only had what was grown in that particular season to choose from. For more information about produce and what season it is grown in, or maybe what you can grow yourself, here is a guide the USDA has available to show you what produce should be available in which seasons: https://snaped.fns.usda.gov/seasonal-produce-guide.

## Cleaning Produce Matters

It may seem silly to you that I have made this subject an individual title. The reason I have done this is because it has value. This is quite a simple process, and one I want you to see for yourself. Not only is it simple, but hopefully will become routine in your home too.

I clean all my produce as soon as I return from the grocery or marketplace, even if some of the produce is not ripe yet. I go through these steps so that it is ready to be enjoyed once the produce is ripe. And if left to do later, it might not get done before my family starts eating it. I even go through the process of washing the produce that gets peeled. It might sound a little extreme, but my grandchildren are very likely to be eating these foods too! I have witnessed too many children dealing with serious health, skin, and even respiratory issues—even cancer. I know I was not present when they sprayed the produce I am buying, so I don't assume that it is clean and free of harmful substances.

Let me also comment on having my veggies cleaned and sliced and in a sealed container ready for when I need a quick snack. Whether my produce is organic or not organic, I go through the process below.

Here is the simple process I use:

- Mix 4 parts water with 1 part lemon juice or vinegar (white or apple cider)
- Soak for 30 to 60 minutes (60 minutes if waxed)
- Scrub with a soft-bristled brush (except berries) under cold running water
- Air or towel dry

# You Can Live Like This

## Citric Acid: it's Not What You Think it Is

In Phase 1, I encourage you to eat none or a minimal amount of canned and processed foods. Processed to me is a deliberate change in the food that occurs before it is packaged. They are not going to just catch a tuna and put it inside a can, right? They need to do something to ready it for canning. The same goes for all processed foods, but some are much more in depth than others. It can be as simple as freezing or drying food to preserve nutrients and freshness or as complex as canning foods, formulating a frozen meal, breakfast cereals, cheeses, bread, creating packaged snacks, convenience foods such as microwaveable meals, cakes, and biscuits, or drinks such as milk, juices, and soft drinks. You can count on the fact that you will find these foods in quick service, fine-dining restaurants, cafeterias, food courts, sports arenas, coffee shops, and other similar locations.

So what does this have to do with citric acid? Let me share that I believe most of us think when we see canned or processed food and the label reads "citric acid" that it is a healthy ingredient. For some of you reading, you may have never even read a food label. You are about to have your eyes opened! We assume that citric acid is an extract from lemon, lime, or other healthy citrus fruit. If you do not see the wording that the citrus acid is from lemon, lime or other citrus fruit, can you be sure that it is? Your guess is as good as mine. I have seen wording saying it is from citrus, and therefore it gives me reason to believe that the others either didn't go to the trouble to state it was from citrus, or it was a lab creation. I suggest to you, that a lab creation may be more popular and less expensive than growing an organic fruit, squeezing it and preserving it in order to add it to foods to help preserve them. If that is the case, then what is the citric acid we are eating and is it good for our bodies?

- Chemical Safety Facts Website (www.chemicalsafetyfacts.org) states that "Citric acid is commonly used as a food additive for natural flavoring and as a preservative." (CFR - Code of Federal Regulations Title 21)
- The U.S. Food and Drug Administration (FDA) states that citric acid is generally recognized as safe (GRAS) as a direct food additive.
- Since the early 1900's, approximately 99 percent of the world's production of manufactured citric acid has been developed from black mold (the Aspergillus niger fungus). Black mold efficiently converts sugars into citric acid. Its fermentation is also generally recognized as safe by the FDA under its Federal Food, Drug, and Cosmetic Act.[8]

This little stroll we just took down Citric Acid Lane gives more information than the food label offers you. And yes, the citric acid is stated to taste like citric acid from fruits we are familiar with. So there you have it. What are the possibilities that the citric acid on the majority of our food labels is lab created, tastes natural, is made from GMO derived products, is a black mold that when fed sugar (that is generally derived from a GMO corn

---

8. The data shared in the three bullets above have been shared by permission, from the ChemicalSafetyFacts.org website and can be found at this link: https://www.accessdata.fda.gov/scripts/cdrh/cfdocs/cfcfr/CFRSearch.cfm?fr=184.1033.

# Chapter 9: Nutritional Balance Defined

starch) is able to convert it into citric acid, and is generally recognized as safe by the FDA—is what is in our foods?

Am I the only one, or do you also recognize that this might not be the natural ingredient you expected to find in your food? I will let you make your own decision on this. If you decide to read labels and be wise about what additives are allowed in your food, you may find yourself feeling better especially in the long run. In following the TEID Lifestyle you are encouraged to keep these additives to a minimum, and go for the real thing.

So let me close this section by saying, it is your choice what goes into your body. Can we do it perfectly? No! But the more we understand and become educated, we are better prepared to choose healthy clean foods. Meaning foods without additives that we can't say or spell. It's just my guess that this will lead to more natural food choices. In other words, be informed and make the best pick from your available choices. Remember, our bodies are looking for variety and balance to support your immune system. In a world where our food is constantly being bombarded with ways to cheapen it's growth, production, and preservation to feed a growing population, learn to make the best choices possible. That is certainly a good start.

I encourage you to make yourself and your family a priority. If you maintain a healthy balance when you eat at home, then you're making great headway. Many families have made some amazing changes with food purchases and style of eating. The result is that these families are reaping the benefits of better choices. You can have these benefits and blessings too.

When you are feeding a young family, why not take the same veggies you're baking and steaming for yourself and puree or mash them for your young ones? Then you also know exactly what they are eating. Shouldn't they get the same balance of healthy nutrients that you're consuming? Of course! Just think of the foundation you are laying for their future health and wellness. Imagine babies and toddlers growing up with strong immune systems and being able to naturally fight off the bad stuff coming against them, especially as they enter school. These children will be ahead of the game. Not to mention they will know what real food tastes like and not battle the crazy food cravings from sugar and packaged snacks that so many kids do today.

You can do this! It just takes a moment to make the decision for good health. This is the beginning of your renewed legacy. What could be more valuable for your family than to inherit a life-long example of healthy balance and being able to live at their optimum weight?

Yes, sometimes there are some surprises in our foods. Let's create foods filled with good surprises—surprises that give life and goodness.

# You Can Live Like This

## Herbs and Spices

By now you may be learning to introduce yourself to using herbs in your recipes. I want to encourage you to try them all at some point, and try them fresh. Dried is good, but fresh is delectable. Just think of the variety of nutrients packed in each one. The flavors available are beyond anything your taste buds have experienced! Using fresh herbs is most likely part of what makes a great chef or culinary enthusiast so popular. Fresh herbs are truly what puts flavor in a meal. You can change a dish up simply by changing up the herbs and spices.

My husband and I grow several herbs and consume them literally every day. We begin each day by adding some to our protein shake. We might add them to a salad at lunch, place them on meat before grilling, or mix them up with our vegetables. Flavor makes our taste buds dance. If we have asparagus, one week I might use thyme and garlic, then the next week I use parsley and oregano. It's never the same dish, which keeps cooking and eating fun and always a new experience. It also makes dining at home and entertaining fun. And not to mention the money that can be saved.

**Katia Shares:**

>When Cindy and I shared our special week together, I learned so many things. Our time was wonderful, and I am still gleaning from all of the experiences we shared. I always love using herbs in my food, but Cindy taught me to mix several of them together. I was more accustomed to using one herb per dish, but using several fresh herbs together brought about an unbelievable flavor to our meals. Every time we sat down to eat, I was so excited to experience the flavors—and, best of all, it was simple and fun. As I look back, all boundaries of what I thought was appropriate to mix together were replaced—out with the old and in with the new! I had a new confidence to try new things. What perfect timing for me.
>
>We made up a soup recipe together one day. We just looked at what vegetables we had and started creating. Not only was it full of fresh, nutritional vegetables and organic bone broth, it was soaring with flavor from all of the fresh herbs and spices that we added—even ginger. Oh, and we topped the soup with a spoonful of chopped Hass avocado. We were like two kids in a toy store as we delightfully prepared our meal together, laughing as we went, and then raved over our own cooking as we ate and cheered each other with "Bon Appétit!"

Here are some safe herbs and spices for those looking for a place to begin:

# Chapter 9: Nutritional Balance Defined

- Basil leaf (sweet)
- Bay leaf
- Chamomile
- Chives
- Cilantro
- Cinnamon
- Cloves
- Dill weed
- Fennel leaf
- Garlic
- Ginger
- Lavender
- Lemon balm
- Mace
- Marjoram leaf
- Onion powder
- Oregano leaf
- Parsley
- Peppermint
- Rosemary
- Saffron
- Sage
- Himalayan pink salt or Celtic sea salt
- Savory leaf
- Spearmint
- Tarragon
- Thyme
- Turmeric

A few points to help get you started:

In broad terms, both herbs and spices come from plants, but herbs are the *fresh* part of the plant while spice is the dried root, dried stalk, seed, or dried fruit of the plant and is almost always *dried,* not fresh. Spices tend to be more potent in flavor than herbs because they are made from crushed portions of plants that are especially rich in essential oils. Herbs can be found fresh or dried, chopped, or whole. Both herbs and spices add flavor; however, herbs are subtle, while spices have a stronger flavor. You can add a small bunch of basil to your pesto, however, you cannot add more than a few peppercorns to it. With spices, less is often more. Herbs and spices can't only be paired with each other, but you can use a combination of two or more herbs or multiple spices.

## Healthy Substitute for Soy Sauce—Coconut Aminos

Coconut aminos is a dark-colored sauce that tastes similar to soy sauce but does not contain soy. It comes from the sap of the coconut plant, not coconuts.

## Sugars and Sugar Substitutes

This tends to be a very confusing subject, somewhat due to the advertisements of those trying to sell processed or fat-free foods. Think about this: wouldn't it be sweet if we could eat sugar without worrying about health consequences? Well, guess what? We can! We just have to choose the right sugar.

Processed sugars can be toxic to the body. They provide nothing but empty calories, and refined sugar is highly addictive, causes blood sugar levels to spike, interferes with nutrient absorption, and even has been linked to contribute to heart disease, weight gain, and other degenerative diseases. But we don't have to live without it.

Swapping out the white stuff for another minimally processed, more natural sugar is better for our bodies. There are alternatives to processed regular sugar that provide some surprising benefits. They are still sugar, but they boast a range of nutrients and health benefits. I literally can picture most of you wiping the sweat from your brow as you expected me to say, "No more sugar of any kind!" But before I type one more word, I need to remind you that it is always about *balance*. So we still need to maintain balance as we consume any of the best sugars.

Sucrose (which is what cane sugar is) and glucose cause insulin levels to spike. Fructose is found in fruit, for the most part, but can also be found in other plants. However, too much fructose can be challenging for the liver to metabolize. If the liver is challenged to metabolize fructose, the liver starts to produce free radicals, one of the many reasons why high-fructose corn syrup is so awful.

## Better Sugars

These include pure maple syrup, coconut nectar, and date syrup. These all score lower on the glycemic index and have lower amounts of fructose. My next choice is local honey.

In essence, what you're looking for in a better sugar is both a low glycemic index, a fructose content that is not too high, and additional nutrients that cane sugar does not offer. When you arrive at Phase 3 and begin to add any form of yogurt, it may be difficult to find one without cane sugar. Remember, if this occurs we are always referring to staying in balance. Therefore, if you reintroduce these, eat them in balance. Which, further defined, is not every meal and not every day; it's just best to limit cane sugar.

**Pure Maple Syrup:** Has low fructose content and therefore a lower glycemic index. Sourced straight from trees and contains minerals, including manganese, riboflavin, zinc, magnesium, and antioxidants. Always confirm the label reads "pure" or you may be getting corn syrup with maple flavoring.

**Coconut Nectar:** Many people are not aware of coconut nectar, so I want to teach what it is. It is the sap collected from the flower blossom of the coconut palm tree. The coconut farmer climbs the tree in the early morning and collects the blossom nectar by slicing the flower. This allows the nectar to flow. The nectar is then watered down and boiled into a syrup consistency. The process is minimal and nothing artificial is added. It boasts high amounts of potassium and electrolytes. Coconut palm sugar is made by crystallization or processing of the coconut flower nectar. So my go-to is coconut nectar because it's one step closer to natural, or one less processing step. And I like the flavor in my baked goods.

**Date Syrup:** It is low on the glycemic index and lower in fructose than most sweeteners. It contains nutrients like magnesium, phosphorus, and zinc. It is also higher in antioxidant properties.

# Chapter 9: Nutritional Balance Defined

**Local Raw Honey:** Honey has amino acids, electrolytes, and antioxidants. It has been touted for its natural antiseptic properties and ability to alleviate allergy symptoms. It does contain a higher fructose level than the others, but is relatively low on the glycemic index.

**Unsulfured Blackstrap Molasses:** Rich in iron, potassium, and calcium. Molasses is a by-product of refined white sugar, and is processed three times to remove as much sucrose as possible. Molasses is categorized by how many times the syrup was boiled and sugar extracted. Molasses is extracted during the first (light), second (dark), or third stage (blackstrap) of boiling. Blackstrap is the darkest, thickest, and most concentrated molasses. The extra boil concentrates the nutrients.

You will notice there are sulfured and unsulfured molasses. The sugarcane used in sulfured molasses does not have as much time to mature, thus the need for preservatives. *Sulfured* means sulfur was added during sugar production to keep the raw sugar cane fresh, kill unwanted bacteria, and whiten the sugar crystals. Unsulfured molasses comes from fully mature sugarcane in which the cane juice is already concentrated. It is also free of sodium dioxide, a preservative and a known allergen.

## Sugar Substitutes

A list of Nonnutritive Sweeteners (NNSs) can be found in this link: https://www.fda.gov/food/food-additives-petitions/additional-information-about-high-intensity-sweeteners-permitted-use-food-united-states.

NNSs are not metabolized in the body and most are generally considered safe for consumption by the FDA. However, there are prevailing concerns over toxicity of "non metabolized" compounds. So if our bodies can not metabolize them, what benefit or, maybe better stated, what side effect do we get from them? For some, the jury is still out. There have been a range of symptoms reported from those consuming NNSs such as headaches, stomachaches and a general ill feeling. Some have questioned if NNSs can actually change the bacterial makeup of your microbiome, throwing gut health out of balance. As we now know, gut health and balance is a very important part of our immune system. Anytime we eat something that is not nutritionally based to feed our body, there will be an increased chance of it affecting us in negative ways and especially increasing inflammation and/or gut permeability. Thus, a few reasons why I have not included NNSs in the TEID Lifestyle.

There is a common point of confusion that I want to clear up. Many think sucralose is sucrose. Sucrose mentioned previously is cane sugar. Sucralose is a NNS.

## Other Sugars not previously mentioned:

**High-Fructose Corn Syrup:** Made through a chemical process that's anything but natural, high-fructose corn syrup is one of the worst offenders for insulin spikes, as it doesn't have to be digested by your body. This stuff actually filters right into your bloodstream and goes wild.

**Agave**: Agave gained notoriety for its low glycemic index, it ultimately was shown to have a higher fructose content than high-fructose corn syrup. It has been marketed as a healthier alternative, but it's really no better than the worst offenders.

**Sugar Alcohols**: like xylitol, erythritol and sorbitol are generally recognized as safe and are commonly in chewing gum and toothpaste because they've been found to protect against tooth decay. They also score low on the glycemic index. While those are both great benefits, the verdict is still out over the side effects on your gut, as they have been found to cause digestive problems. The problem is that your body can't digest most sugar alcohols, so they travel to the large intestine, where they are metabolized by gut bacteria. If you eat a lot of sugar alcohols in a short period of time, it can lead to gas, bloating, and diarrhea. The biggest offenders are sorbitol and maltitol.

## The Nutrition Facts Label

After twenty years of not being updated, the nutrition facts label has been updated.

### The new label must now include the following:
- Total fat
- Saturated fat
- Trans fat
- Cholesterol
- Sodium
- Total carbohydrate
- Dietary fiber
- Total sugars
- Added sugars
- Protein
- Certain vitamins and minerals may be listed voluntarily

Labels no longer reflect portion sizes based on what Americans should eat or drink but instead on what they actually consume. For instance, the serving size for soda went from 8 ounces to 12 ounces, and a serving of yogurt went from 8 ounces to 6 ounces.

### Additional changes include:
- Servings sizes and calories printed in a larger, bold font.
- Dual columns (on some products) with the nutritional information for a single serving in one column, and for the entire package in the other column.
- Updated daily values.
- Nutrient information for vitamin D, potassium, and added sugars.

## Chapter 9: Nutritional Balance Defined

- No more calories from fat. Science shows that the type of fat is more important than the amount of fat. Switching to good fats may help lower your blood pressure and prevent heart disease.

These updates were made according to the FDA to promote awareness, increase usage of nutritional information and guidelines, and help consumers make healthier choices by:

- Choosing items that are high in fiber, vitamins and minerals, and lower in saturated fat, trans fat, sodium, and added sugars.
- Comparing serving sizes on items to make sure you're looking at nutrition facts for similar portions.
- Checking the calories on nutrition labels and adjusting your intake based on your health care provider's advice.
- Giving a better understanding of the percentages of daily values.

**The Research behind the Change**

Science played a big role in the new label. For example, according to the National Academies of Sciences, Engineering and Medicine's *Dietary Reference Intakes for Sodium and Potassium* report, getting more potassium may lower blood pressure. Vitamin D helps your body absorb calcium and is critical for bone health. It is also associated with an increased risk of chronic disease. Both vitamin D and potassium are nutrients that Americans don't get enough of. The FDA also dropped nutrients from the new label. It now no longer requires vitamins A and C to be listed because Americans are rarely deficient in these. And the "added sugars" entry on the new label because, based on studies, food choices based on added sugars could prevent over 350,000 cases of heart disease and close to 600,000 cases of diabetes over twenty years.

The FDA recommends Americans get the daily values (DV) of nutrients to achieve optimal health. The percentage of daily values is listed on Nutrition Facts labels, but they can be hard to interpret. Here's an easy way to use them. In a nutshell, if a food serving has 5% or less of the DV of a nutrient, it's considered low in that nutrient. If a food serving has 20% or more of the DV of a nutrient, it's considered high in that nutrient. On nutrition facts labels, look for the column marked "% Daily Value." If you want to get more vitamin D from your diet, reach for foods with 20% or more of the recommended DV. If, on the other hand, you want to consume less sodium, find foods with 5% or less of the recommended DV.[9]

**Important Points to Remember When Reading Nutrition Facts Label Ingredients**

The ingredients are listed in order of predominance, with the ingredients used in the greatest amount first, followed in descending order by those in smaller amounts. The label must list the names of any FDA-certified color additives (e.g., FD&C Blue No. 1 or the abbreviated name, Blue 1).[10]

---

9. For more information, see https://www.fda.gov/food/food-labeling-nutrition/changes-nutrition-facts-label
10. Ibid.

- When you see a product and the first item listed is water, think about what you are paying for as you do a product comparison.
- When choosing to follow the TEID Lifestyle, it is very helpful to read this ingredient list and see what good fats and what bad fats are included and remembering the order of placement is valuable too. Choose the good fats.
- We often read the highlights on the package and automatically believe when it is called heart-healthy, natural, or just good for you. Now you are equipped to read the Nutrition Facts Label, but don't stop there. Keep reading through the ingredient list to confirm that the product lines up with what you consider to be healthy, heart-healthy, natural, or balanced.
- Do your own experiment on foods that are your go-to. For example, I pick up a bag of regular chips/snacks and see bad fats. Then I pick up a bag of chips/snacks that state they are fat-free. They have additives I would not normally eat, cannot pronounce, or have added artificial sugars. Finally, I look at chips/snacks made in avocado oil and notice there is a big difference in the goodness of this product made with healthy fats.
- When you notice there are dyes included in the product (from pickles/relish to kid's snacks and candies), it is important that you know if the dye is safe or not.
- Many times if you do a comparison, you can find a product with just the ingredients you are looking for. For example, tuna can be just tuna, or it can have additives and/or preservatives. Frozen shrimp can be just wild shrimp or it can be wild shrimp with preservatives. Make it your goal to choose food without the extra additives when available.
- There are many sugars and artificial sugars being added to our foods, especially snacks or fat-free foods today. It may have been better for you to eat the regular item.
- Flavorings are just that. A flavoring that has been added. We usually assume this is good for us. Flavorings can be made from almost anything (remember citrus flavors).
- If you are gluten free, you are looking for the gluten-free flours, and not a lot of bad additives.
- Summary: you are looking to see what is in a product and determine if it has hidden items you would rather not eat or is filled with a good, healthy balance. Remember, flours, dyes, additives, preservatives, fats, sugars, artificial anythings, fillers, etc. all affect your health for better or worse. It pays to read the labels.

Know your body. Know your health. Set some goals and make the best choices you can make. Your body will thank you for years to come!

# Chapter 10

# NUTRITION BEGINS AT HOME

We have so much information at our fingertips today compared to any other time in history. There is really no excuse not to be knowledgeable or to educate ourselves, except for the busyness of life. If you only take a few minutes a day, you will be surprised what a difference this can make at the end of one year, two years, and so on. It will literally change your life!

This book is not only meant to be a guide for you but an inspiration. I pray you are ready to take charge of your life and health after this reading. Just take one small step a day to equip yourself further. If you have family at home with you, you are so blessed to have this information at your fingertips. Now you have the opportunity to influence their lives too. America currently has more unhealthy and obese children than ever before. You are privileged to share by your attitude and your actions with those around you. This is so much more powerful than you can imagine! Just by making a choice for your health and becoming balanced, you are impacting your family. Those watching closely will also learn how to avoid future health issues by making healthy choices. I have learned that it can literally save lives—emotionally and physically—as we spread hope and knowledge. Blessings to you for not only taking charge of your life but for spreading health and longevity. If no one has told you today, let me say it, "You are amazing!" Allow yourself the freedom to walk into your new lifestyle with confidence.

### Meal Planning and Shopping Simplified

This section could be a book all by itself. To keep it simple, I will drop some very important key points here and let you run with them. My sister Sandi added some points in this chapter too. I pray you will be encouraged to create your own plan of action with the inspiration we hope to drip on you.

# You Can Live Like This

**From Sandi:**

> First of all, I sit down with paper and pen and begin to plan my meals for the week. I like to have variety in our meals. I love trying new recipes but tend to go for the faster and easier recipes. My family has a few favorite ones, so they get on our menu more often. I usually make sure my meals for the weekend are fun, maybe something that we would order out in a restaurant. I also plan our lunches. I like to pack my lunch. I laugh at myself when I tell my husband that he can't buy lunches as good as I pack for him. Yes, I know it is fun to go out to eat once in a while, and we do.
>
> My favorite time to shop is first thing in the morning when the store is opening. I usually have my protein shake on my way to the store. I also use this trick when we are going out to eat, dining with friends, or going to a party. Instead of having my shake for breakfast, I switch it up and save it for my pre-outing meal. If my tummy is content, then I am sure to make better choices, which results in a happier me when I step on the scale the morning after.
>
> There are so many options today for grocery shopping. My daughter does all of her grocery shopping online for pickup. Do whatever fits your lifestyle and your budget! When I head into the store, I stay in the outside aisles of the store. Believe me, there's nothing up and down all those interior isles that will make me feel healthy or good about myself. Giving my family healthy options is the very best thing I can do for them. Yes, they might fuss at first but stay *strong*, you will be glad very soon that you have joined this lifestyle too!

I don't have a specific day when I plan my meals. It depends on when we run out of food. I try hard not to go grocery shopping on the weekends. I would rather play on those days. I love fresh produce so I try to keep some go-to produce, on the counter or in our refrigerator at all times. I love having meals full of variety. And like Sandi, I love to try new ideas. I often read the recipe and do it my way. When I find a good meal while dining out, I love to try and recreate the recipe at home my way. If we have leftovers, I just hold them for a few days before doing a rerun, thus two meals were just prepared instead of one. We eat almost all fresh vegetables. It is rare for me to buy a frozen vegetable, and almost never canned vegetables. They just don't taste or look the same to me.

I love to prepare my meals with *pizzazz*! In other words, I like it to look like something we would get when dining out. It is fun, and when I create a sweet or romantic ambiance, the food seems to taste better too. I even like doing this with my grandchildren. Even though I stay busy, I don't do grocery ordering and pickup or delivery routinely. But I know it makes life easier for one of my daughters-in-law while taxiing three kiddos to and from school and covering work and all of her responsibilities. Remember, it is always an option if you're short on time.

My menu and grocery list is on my phone. I like to use an app like Out of Milk or Anylist to keep my grocery list up to date and my meal plan at my fingertips. What is great about the Anylist app is that my husband and I share the app, so either one of us can make entries or cross it off of the

## Chapter 10: Nutrition Begins at Home

list while shopping. There are many apps to choose from, so find one that works for you if you need simplification.

Whenever I have to chop and dice in meal preparation, I love to include my husband. He is much better at this than I am. When I'm working, I like to have something prepared so when I walk in the door, I can pop it into the oven, into the air fryer, or on the grill. I might prepare it early in the morning or the night prior while we are doing dinner clean-up. Or maybe it will be a salad night with leftover beef, chicken, or fish with a bite of fruit. We don't use a microwave, so we heat everything in the oven or air-fryer. It is just as simple once you get used to it. Sometimes I even pull the crockpot out and get it going before leaving in the morning. Then we come home and can just eat without waiting on the food to cook. Let me make a comment here. If I'm hungry, I will have a plate of fresh veggies ready to munch on. That keeps me from grazing on the meal while I am preparing it.

Here are a few more tips about meal planning and grocery shopping:

- Print out the phase you are in and keep it on you at all times, especially in the grocery store or when dining out.
- Planning out your weekly meals and combining them to your grocery list can save money. This means looking at the recipes to be sure you listed all of the ingredients you need.
- Having a grocery list and sticking to it keeps unwanted foods from coming home with you. You will be amazed at how quickly you will find the healthy choices have so much more flavor than you ever realized. They are so much better for you than some of your old choices.
- If you have kids, shopping alone whenever possible might keep some temptations from coming home with you, thus spending more money than planned.
- On the other hand, meal planning is a great way to include older children and teach them about meal planning, nutrition, variety, grocery shopping, budgeting, preparation, and cooking.
- Meal planning makes this lifestyle transition easier and more fun.
- **Never go to the grocery store hungry!** Have a healthy snack before heading inside.
- If you have more than one store to choose from, check the ads first. Then you are sure to get the best buy for your dollar. Some, like Sandi, will hit more than one store. Remember, she goes first thing in the morning before her day has gotten away from her. Others may need to go when convenient, and every day might be different. You may need to keep it simple by going to one store, so it might be necessary to change the meal plan to accommodate what is available at that store. It might mean you need to have a few extra meals on the list to choose from if this dilemma strikes.
- As you go into the store, remember it's the outside aisles that have the real food.
- If you have family or friends over and they bring food or goodies with them that are not on your phase, make sure the food goes home with them when they leave, take it to work with you and share it, or send it with your husband to the lunchroom at his work; find a way to re-gift it. You are allowed to bless others and set boundaries to protect yourself.

# You Can Live Like This

## Ways to Include Your Family

I want to encourage you to bring this blessing of health home to your family. Studies have shown that there is a definite link between one's overall wellbeing and nutritious meals. Keep in mind that poor nutrition leads to inflammation, and inflammation is a forerunner to our health and immune system weakening. I hope you see this as a privilege to teach your family by example and include them so they can learn too.

Today more than ever, children are also struggling or dealing with stress. We know good wellbeing is vitally important. It is amazing what having a healthy emotional outlook can make and how it can affect many areas of our children's lives too. So let's talk about some ways to include your family and help them feel good.

Kids can be picky eaters, but just like adults, there might be some foods they don't want because they just don't agree with their little tummy. Maybe they don't like dairy; it might be because they get gastrointestinal discomfort after eating it. So give choices and let them have a part in planning the week's menu. Maybe they can plan one dinner and even help prepare it, or write out the grocery list for you. They could cross the items off of the list while shopping, even if in the grocery cart. Have them help you check the pantry for ingredients. Let them make a list of some of their favorite foods or meals. You can always arrange and adjust their ideas to make the meal healthy. Have them clip coupons for you. Maybe they can create a meal calendar for the week and hang it on the refrigerator, so everyone is on the same page. Perhaps they can help prepare a fruit salad or another healthy snack to put in the refrigerator for an after-school snack.

As you are learning to read the label and check out the ingredients, especially for those unwanted hidden surprises, teach your children how to do it too. You will get to the point where you have helpers everywhere, which will eventually be a huge blessing in your home, and at the same time, they are learning how to be healthy for life. Encourage kids to set the table or even make centerpieces, napkin holders, name cards, or placemats. Kids love doing art, and getting their creative juices flowing can add fun to their task. This will build their confidence and can go a long way for joy-filled discussions during meals. Don't make them have to do it your way or perfectly. Let them be kids.

When kids are involved in choosing the menu or preparing the food, there is a completely different atmosphere around the dinner table than when they sat down to something they didn't like or weren't in the mood for. Lastly, I cannot encourage you enough to get back to family dinners at least a few nights a week. This is critical while kids are growing up! It gives them a place to belong, call home, and learn many things, including manners, etiquette, responsibility, communication, and creativity. Keep meal times light and fun!

# Chapter 10: Nutrition Begins at Home

## Phase I: Sample Menu for Seven Days

*This is only a sample for Phase 1, your first 30-60 days. Then Phase 2 will include the additions found in the Phase 2 chart. Phase 3 will include the additions you will add to Phase 2 following Reintroduction.*

All items included in the menu below go along with the guidelines (organic, grass-fed, without sugar, etc.) in this book, even if not shown here. Remember to use the guidelines from Chapter 5 to determine your amounts. If you prefer to use the protein shake for a meal other than breakfast, that works too. This is only a sample, so please feel free if you want to substitute other meats, vegetables, or fat found in the Phase 1 "EAT" column. If you are not a seafood lover, this is a great opportunity to give it another try. This sample menu is only to give you a place to begin. Maybe add the coconut aminos to the dish. Plan to be creative with your combinations and enjoy this journey.

I loved keeping a bowl of cut-up crunchy veggies in the fridge when I began. When snack time came, I could just dish up and add my salad dressing mixture (below), yeast granules, and herbs, an olive or two, and my snack was complete.

While preparing meals, it is not uncommon for me to plan a little extra for a snack in a day or two that I place in a sealed container. Then I pull it out when I run short on time.

Because all of my produce is already cleaned and in a colander in the fridge, I can easily grab a spoonful to add to my snack or meal. My celery and other veggies are also cleaned and in a container, ready to be added to a snack or a meal.

Taking the time to have your produce clean and ready makes a huge difference when you are running short on time and want to stay on track. The preparation we talked about earlier gives you the ability to win.

## DAY 1

**Breakfast:**
- Protein shake, as per choices in Chapter 8

**Snack:**
- 8 oz organic bone broth
- Organic apple

**Lunch:**
- Salad with chopped veggies, ½ avocado, organic chicken, kiwi
- Homemade dressing: 2 parts avocado oil or organic extra virgin olive oil to 1 part red wine vinegar, white wine vinegar or coconut vinegar (vinegars without sugar)

**Snack:**
- Olives
- Celery sticks

**Dinner:**
- Wild tuna, lightly pan-seared
- Zucchini sautéed in oil with onion
- Organic berry salad with mint

**Bedtime Snack:**
- Hot herbal decaf tea
- A bite of meat wrapped in a lettuce leaf with a pickle (no sugar added)

## DAY 2

**Breakfast:**
- Protein shake

**Snack:**
- Cucumber slices with mashed Hass avocado with garlic and onion and lime/lemon squeeze

**Lunch:**
- Spinach salad with fresh herbs topped with a few organic fresh blackberries served with sliced steak (organic grass-fed and grass-finished)
- Homemade dressing: 2 parts avocado oil or organic extra virgin olive oil to 1 part red wine vinegar, white wine vinegar, or coconut vinegar (vinegars without sugar), warmed and drizzled over it all

**Snack:**
- Pink grapefruit
- Cauliflower florets
- Olives

**Dinner:**
- Soup made with organic bone broth (with or without meat) vegetables of choice, fresh herbs, and topped with chunks of avocado

**Bedtime Snack:**
- 4-8 ounces organic bone broth
- Celery sticks

## CHAPTER 10: NUTRITION BEGINS AT HOME

| DAY 3 | |
|---|---|
| **Breakfast:**<br>• Protein shake<br>**Snack:**<br>• ½ Hass avocado, purple onion, and cilantro. All chopped and drizzled in lime juice. Serve with vegetable slices<br>**Lunch:**<br>• Shrimp cold or sautéed in oil of your choice, chopped organic English cucumber, and onion with fresh thyme or other herbs, small organic orange, or other fruit.<br>• All drizzled with coconut aminos | **Snack:**<br>• Olives<br>• Celery sticks<br>**Dinner:**<br>• Grilled organic grass-fed/grass-finished beef or bison burger with heavy lettuce wrap, pickle (no sugar added), onion, herbs, and drizzled with coconut aminos<br>• A cup of organic fruit<br>**Bedtime Snack:**<br>• A small cup of the soup from Day 2 |

| DAY 4 | |
|---|---|
| **Breakfast:**<br>• Protein shake<br>**Snack:**<br>• ½ cup of wild albacore tuna (may have extra virgin olive oil added if in the can) serve on a lettuce leaf with a pickle (no sugar added)<br>**Lunch:**<br>• Grilled, baked, or air-fried chicken<br>• Brussels sprouts drizzled in oil and herbs. Cook side by side.<br>• All can be drizzled with lemon juice or coconut aminos.<br>• A small bowl of organic strawberries | **Snack:**<br>• 4-8 ounces organic bone broth topped with chopped avocado and yeast granules/flakes<br>**Dinner:**<br>• Wild Salmon drizzled with coconut aminos<br>• Roasted asparagus with herbs<br>• Mashed cauliflower with teaspoon ghee and sprigs of parsley<br>• Kiwi chopped<br>**Bedtime Snack:**<br>• Herbal decaf tea<br>• A bite of chicken wrapped in a lettuce leaf |

## DAY 5

**Breakfast:**
- Protein shake

**Snack:**
- Cucumber slices with mashed Hass avocado with garlic and onion and lime/lemon squeeze

**Lunch:**
- Roasted organic turkey
- ½ white sweet potato or ½ regular sweet potato
- Chopped organic salad of organic celery, onion, radish, and dressing or coconut aminos

**Snack:**
- Grapefruit
- Bowl of salad greens with oil and vinegar

**Dinner:**
- Grilled seafood (or a meat of your choice) with fresh herbs, lemon or lime, and oil
- Steamed or roasted carrot, broccoli, and cauliflower mixed
- Organic unsweetened applesauce with cinnamon.

**Bedtime Snack:**
- Small organic fruit
- ¼ avocado
- Herbal decaf tea

## DAY 6

**Breakfast:**
- Protein shake

**Snack:**
- Organic fruit
- Olives

**Lunch:**
- Ground organic cooked meat, oil, freshly grated ginger, a sprinkle of cinnamon, with herbs on top or chunks of apple, wrapped in cabbage leaves and baked

**Snack:**
- ½ cup of wild albacore tuna (may have extra virgin olive oil added if in the can) serve on a lettuce leaf with a pickle (no sugar added)

**Dinner:**
- Steak (organic grass-fed and grass-finished)
- Broccolini
- Mixed berry salad

**Bedtime Snack:**
- Organic bone broth 4-8 ounces
- ¼ avocado with a lime squeeze

# Chapter 10: Nutrition Begins at Home

| DAY 7 | |
|---|---|
| **Breakfast:**<br>• Protein shake<br>**Snack:**<br>• Cucumber slices with mashed sardine topped with lemon/lime slices<br>**Lunch:**<br>• Baked butternut squash (¼-½) or riced cauliflower<br>• Sautéed scallops drizzled in coconut aminos<br>• Small bowl of organic berries | **Snack:**<br>• Small piece of cabbage roll from Day 6<br>**Dinner:**<br>• Grilled pork<br>• Okra roasted in air-fryer, sauerkraut (without sugar), or mashed chiquote topped with chives/ghee<br>• A small bowl of fruit.<br>**Bedtime Snack:**<br>• Organic fruit<br>• ¼ avocado<br>• Herbal decaf hot tea |

## Micro-Greens You Can Grow at Home

This happens to be one of my very favorite subjects! My husband and I started growing micro-greens when we read that they can contain up to forty times the nutrients of regular store bought vegetables. And the fact is, that my husband is totally in his element when he is "playing in the dirt." He was privileged to grow up in a rural area where having animals and a garden was the norm. His grandparents farmed his family's land for many years. They grew various types of produce and carried it to the farmers market to sell at harvest. My husband was always by their side, whether in the fields or at the market. What I had to learn about growing things and the beauty of reaping the blessings of your harvest, my husband got naturally from his childhood experiences. Later, his family got into raising cattle, and his knowledge of raising a healthy, happy animal and the importance of taking care of your food and its food sources has been invaluable for our family.

Here is a little lesson in growing micro-greens at home that we created for our family and friends. After getting started, I purchased a little greenhouse for my husband's birthday. He has had so much enjoyment growing our micro-greens on our back deck. It's his little piece of heaven on earth.

**Sunflower Micro-Greens**

Our story began by purchasing our sunflower micro-greens from the same local farmer we also got our grass-fed beef. When we called to place our next order, he informed us that he could not keep enough greens to supply us for the next few weeks due to interest from his local community. So we decided to grow our own. Before this, we had only played with growing some sprouts, so this was to be a new adventure. We ordered our organic, non-GMO, black oil sunflower seeds online.

We began small by going to the local department store to get a couple of trays.

We bought plain potting soil in a bag (not garden or fertilized soil).

Our Process:

- Soak 1½ cup of organic sunflower seeds in a bowl of tap water for eight hours
- Placed them on top of the soil
- Cover with enough soil to lightly cover them
- Do not fill all of the trays the first day if you want to plant them in stages

Thus the growing process began: Day 1:

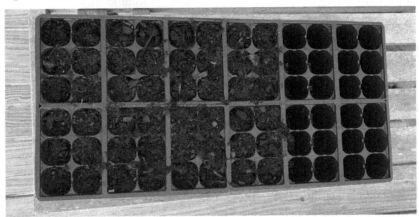

**Note**: bring potting soil up to the top edge of each container so you can snip at the top of the tray line when mature.

Mist them once a day with a spray bottle filled with water (mist enough to keep them moist but not saturated). As they begin to push their way through the soil they might throw a little soil out on the surrounding area.

# Chapter 10: Nutrition Begins at Home

Sneak peek: Day 3:

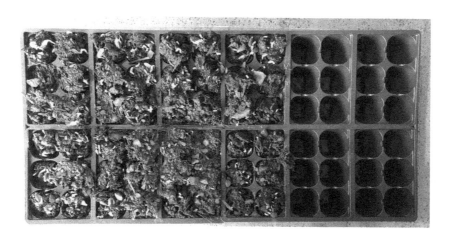

If it's hot outside, they will dry out quicker and may need more misting. If it is cold, you may need to bring them inside or cover them for protection.

Day 5:

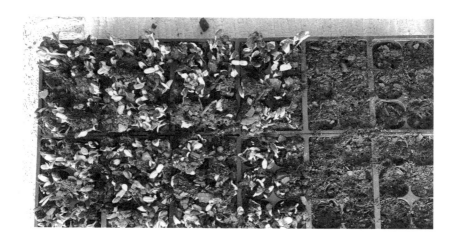

With each new day, you will see new growth.

Day 7:

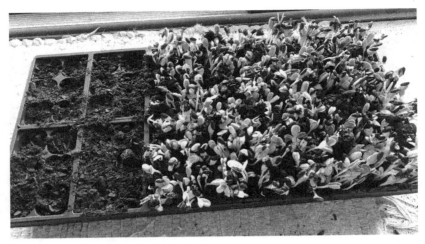

Around day 10, you will have something that looks like this. As you see, I already snipped a few because I had the munchies.

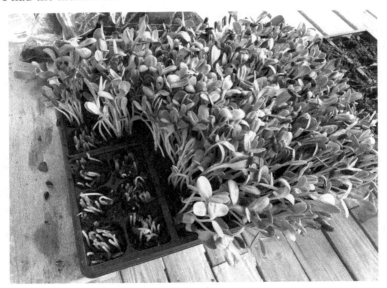

And now the real taste test begins. Cut them and pull off the seedpods. Then store in a sealed container in the refrigerator. When you are ready to use, just wash, dry, and eat.

It is now time to enjoy your micro-greens in a salad or a lettuce wrap. The sky's the limit! I sometimes just munch on them alone. They are so delicious and nutritious. Our grandchildren love eating them too. This can be a great family project to learn about the principles of seeding, planting, and enjoying the bounty of your harvest!

## Chapter 10: Nutrition Begins at Home

Day 10:

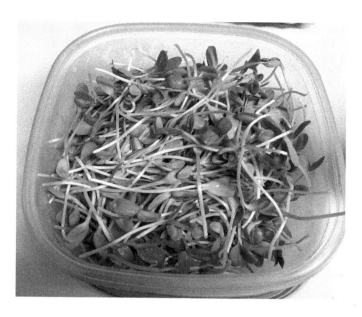

**Health Benefits of Sunflower Micro-Greens:**
- A perfect source of complete protein. They are considered to be the most balanced of all of the sources of essential amino acids, helping to repair muscle tissue and aid in enzymatic functions in the body.
- Help build our skeletal, muscular, and neurological systems.
- Activate every cell of the immune system and help to keep gut bacteria healthy and balanced, thus improving our ability to fight disease.
- Boost fertility as they contain high amounts of zinc.
- They are a nutritional powerhouse packed with vitamins A, B complex, D, and E; they also contain calcium, copper, iron, magnesium, potassium, and phosphorus.
- Rich in chlorophyll, which benefits many functions within the body, including building blood supply, revitalizing tissue, calming inflammation, activating enzymes, and deodorizing the body.
- Boosts antioxidant capacity and is high in nutrition.

The next step for us was to learn about the plethora of micro-greens we could grow. This led to us experimenting with many more. Here are a few of our favorites:

- Broccoli
- Radish
- Kohlrabi
- Lettuce
- Arugula

- Beets
- Cabbage
- Cauliflower

Space is not an issue for growing micro-greens. You can even place them inside at a sunny window. You don't have to have a greenhouse. You don't have to have a green thumb. It's pretty simple, and there are no weeds and no bugs. You only wait a very short time to enjoy the bounty of your harvest. When you think about the amount of nutrients you are getting, it is worth the learning curve if you have never gardened before.

We purchase our seeds in bulk and buy organic when available. If you were to purchase these micro-greens from a market, you would pay around $2.00/ounce. The seeds, soil, and trays (which you can use over and over) are a fraction of the cost. You might even get creative and save your kitchen scraps and compost them. This makes for healthy soil. My husband adds a little organic fertilizer to his composted soil to help the micro-greens green-up. We have made a whole salad out of micro-greens. It is amazing all of the flavors you will find in a variety of micro-greens, some nutty, some spicy, some mild, some stronger, and some like raw veggies.

# Chapter 11

## IF THESE CAN DO IT, SO CAN YOU!

Too many people overestimate what they can do in a day but underestimate what they can do in a few months or a year. Listen to the testimonies of these committed individuals.

### Gina Merritt

I am a sixty-year-old mother of four grown children. I retired as a flight attendant after twenty-five years. Most of my career I was required to have a bi-annual review, which included a weight check. Yes, getting on a scale in front of co-workers and supervisors—even after having each of my babies. No need to say anymore! I'm sharing to give you *hope*. For many years I struggled with staying at a healthy body weight. I lost count of how many diets and programs I tried and failed at. I also lost count of the dollars I spent on books, programs, classes, and remedies. I'm so forever grateful for what the TEID Lifestyle has given me! Being the recipient of Cindy's knowledge, wisdom, patience, and encouragement along this wonderful journey allowed me to finally succeed. The frustration I felt before I was introduced to this balanced lifestyle is gone. I will never look again for a program or a diet. This is the vehicle I had been praying to find.

My entire family, including my grandchildren, can and are following this lifestyle. This is for everyone, even if you do not need to shed pounds. The education and confidence I gleaned are priceless! She taught me so much about my body, how it works, how food works, what is good food, and what is not best. And all of this happened in such a short time. I never received this kind of education and knowledge through all of the dollars I spent, nor did I gain confidence in myself. My entire body has taken a complete turn; I even look younger.

When I began, I was twenty pounds overweight. I began to have health issues, including thyroid imbalance and auto-immune disease symptoms. I wasn't sleeping well and often felt tired. Through the TEID Lifestyle, I lost twenty pounds over four months and have maintained my weight and healthy balance. I always regained the weight several months later on all of the other programs. I will be honest; even when I get off track a little bit, I can get back on track quickly and have maintained my goal weight.

I have so much energy. I sleep better. My confidence is through the roof, and my blood work results are almost all in a normal range. Woo-hoo! That alone is a blessing. My doctors are asking me what I am doing. They love my results and want to endorse this lifestyle. We were desperately searching when we found out that my sister had created the TEID Lifestyle. She also educated my husband, who was dealing with some major health issues, as well as healing his body from three major surgeries in one year. All of our children, including our sons-in-law, were able to obtain this healthy balance and also shed the extra pounds. We all feel amazing and have improved energy. My husband dropped thirty-eight pounds and feels a hundred percent better. The TEID Lifestyle has guided us back to our hot and healthy bodies.

This works—walk away from your doubt! We did. And I am so thankful that we now know how to live life to the fullest. It gives us peace of mind to know we are taking responsibility for our health. This will also decrease our chances of being a burden to our children as we age.

Thank you, Cindy, for following your passion. We, too, want to tell everyone that *you can live life to the fullest!*

## Katia Oliveira

I don't want to share my past of ups and downs that created so many bad habits in me. In my case, compulsive overeating was my behavior. I realize now that I was overeating to hide, or you could say to protect myself, from the emotional pain I was carrying.

God provided me with a full week with my dear friend in paradise (Marathon, Florida Keys). I had no idea that my life was about to change radically as we spent an entire week together.

I opened up and shared all of the frustrations that I was carrying. These things had messed with my emotions and had stolen my peace. Whatever balance I might have had early in my life was sucked out of me. That week, she not only listened to me and prayed with me as my friend, but she also taught me what healthy balance and eating well look like. This began a new journey for me. I was able to forgive not only the people who had hurt me, but most importantly, I was able to forgive myself! My peace and love for myself returned and continue to grow.

That week while I was learning, I didn't do everything the way she was teaching me. I wanted to take my time letting go and putting both feet into the water. Even so, as my peace began to return, I knew I was in a new place. To my excitement, I still lost four pounds. In one month, I lost sixteen pounds and already felt great. I feel confident in myself. And what I thought was my worst enemy—the scale—had become my best friend.

Thank you, Cindy, for being there for me and bringing back my sunshine.

## CHAPTER 11: IF THESE CAN DO IT, SO CAN YOU!

Update after one year: I have now lost fifty-five pounds. Last month, I celebrated four family birthdays and confidently danced my way through the month. Yes, I gained a pound or two, but it was off quickly. Others are noticing and asking what I am doing. I love sharing, and I love the new me!

**BEFORE**            **AFTER**

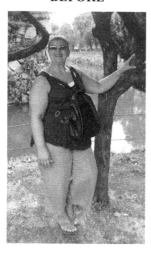 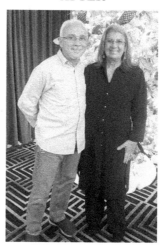

### Steve Merritt

I am fifty-nine years old and a retired pro barefoot water skier. After competing for over twenty years and being the best on the water, I put my body through many injuries, which caused me to have many surgeries in my older years. I've had surgery on my wrist, both lower arms, both hips have had total hip replacements, both shoulders total reconstruction, hernia and neck surgery, to mention a few.

In May of 2016, I woke up with my right arm paralyzed. It was a huge health scare for me. I went to a heart doctor because I had stroke-like symptoms. The doctor said something was going on with the nerves in my neck, which led to my last surgery. I thought I was pretty healthy, but my body had gone through so much after having all of these surgeries. I was introduced to Cindy's program while facing these health challenges.

As I got educated, I realized I was very unhealthy and needed something to help me drop excess weight and help in my body's healing process. Since following the TEID Lifestyle, my body is healing, and I really feel like a different person. The results I have seen and felt are just amazing. I am down thirty-eight pounds, I sleep better with no more snoring, my skin no longer shows symptoms of eczema, there are no little aches and pains, I'm healing faster, and my paralyzed arm; well, let me tell you that I am now up to handling eight pounds of weight, which is a miracle. The doctor told me I might never get my arm back. I feel that with healing my leaky gut, eating proper nutrition, and losing my excess weight, my body is now back and able to fight like the old me would have.

I am thankful to Cindy for sharing her knowledge. What I have learned about health and balance is helping me take my body to a level I did not see possible. My entire family follows the TEID Lifestyle, including our grandchildren. I have even learned how to shop for food, prepare food, know when to eat, what to eat, and how to balance portions in my meals. I often travel for business, and now I know I can live this way, anywhere I am—and so can you.

I have always been on some sort of a diet but never had results such as this. I'm never hungry. That's huge! I'm a prime example. I looked strong and healthy, but I was very unhealthy. One of the best things is that Cindy explains the little details and the big details too. This has been worth millions to me. We are thankful for all we have learned. It is not always easy to share your story with the world, but I share mine to let you know you can be healthy and live a long healthy life, just like God intended for you to live.

## Mia Whitt

I am a thirty-four-year-old mom of three. I have been on some kind of program as well as in many sports to keep my weight off for as long as I can remember. I always felt my battle with weight was due to being short. After being introduced to the TEID Lifestyle, I now realize it was really about my choices. I now know how to choose healthy food and balance and can step off of the roller coaster ride I have been on for years. I introduced this lifestyle to my husband and children just by including these principles in our everyday lives.

I have learned so much from Cindy. I now understand the importance of meal prepping, creating a balance of food choices for my family, portions, and what foods are best for my body, especially when it comes to revving up my metabolism. I have lost excess body weight up to twenty-five pounds, even the baby weight I was still carrying. And, by the way, during my last pregnancy, I was able to control my blood sugar with my food choices after my diagnosis of gestational diabetes. While living this lifestyle, I know I can continue to be balanced and maintain my weight, even as we grow our family. I am delighted to share that I have more energy. This is huge, as I still get up with toddlers at night. I have been accustomed to living on coffee to help me through the day, but not anymore! My skin was dry, but now it feels amazing. My hormones went into a normal range, which is a total blessing for my husband and me. I no longer have night sweats, which have always been an issue after the birth of every child, and never improved until now. That alone is huge.

Now for my oldest child, I had to give him over-the-counter and then eventually prescribed medication every day to have a daily bowel movement. I knew the medications were not something I should give him every day, but at the time, I had no other choice until I was introduced to this lifestyle and healthy balance. Now he eats nutritionally and has regular daily bowel movements, sometimes even two a day. He seemed very hyper. He now eats balanced meals of foods that he loves, and we see a huge difference in his personality and behavior. He also had eczema behind his

# Chapter 11: If These Can Do it, So Can You!

knees, which bothered him and was very itchy. It cleared up approximately two weeks after the change in his diet.

My second child loves everything I feed him now and has done amazing in this transition. My husband got on board too. He wanted to lose belly fat, and has lost twenty pounds. He also had migraines weekly and they have since disappeared by changing his way of eating.

It's really quite simple. We just print out the phase we are in and follow it. If it is on the "EAT" list, we eat it. Now that my husband has learned some basics, he even packs his lunch and can stay on target all day while he is working. If you read between the lines of my story, you will notice that we looked good from the outside, but we were falling apart on the inside. Our bodies were not functioning as God had intended. Thank you, Cindy, for your knowledge, time, and wisdom. We all feel amazing!

## Raimi Rutledge

I am a mother of a toddler and an infant, and am a retired professional wakeboarder. My biggest problem with losing weight was always about trying to be consistent. I found it difficult to stick to a diet or program when I was always hungry. I tried many different diets, including cutting back on calories in my diet. I had spent many hours daily training in the gym and on the water in my career. I was burning a lot of calories, so not eating much because I was always trying to cut calories was very frustrating. I was starving all the time and all I thought about was food. I spent the last few years of my career in that cycle and had no energy.

After transitioning into the TEID Lifestyle, I realized it was a lot easier to eat however much I wanted, and I now know what are good choices for my body. What a great learning curve and huge step forward this has been for me! I learned a lot about different foods and what we need to put in our bodies to lose weight and feel good. After competing over ten years as a professional athlete, I had many injuries. My biggest injury was two herniated discs in my lower back that are so painful that I can barely walk at times. Eating better and losing that extra weight I was carrying around has taken that pain away almost completely! I feel better physically and I'm more confident with myself now than I was before.

I also noticed a difference in my energy level just two weeks after I began. I was very tired all the time before, and now I'm ready for everything! After the first week, I couldn't help but notice the difference on the scale. I also felt improvement physically and emotionally. Those were my two main goals! I knew it was going to get even better from there. My lifestyle has definitely changed from my old ways. The change is so easy to maintain.

My husband, Bradlee, wasn't a fan of going to the gym, nor was he involved at a professional level of training as I was. As we were learning the TEID Lifestyle, he realized that he didn't have much of a nutritional foundation. This motivated us, and now we have one more thing to enjoy together as a family. We are raising our son to make good choices. We are now eating healthy while on the road traveling or going out to dinner. When at home, we have learned to get creative and make it fun. We love the changes we have made and would definitely encourage others to make a choice to improve their lives through the TEID Lifestyle!

## Mindy Miller

I am a wife, mom, and working professional. I didn't really struggle with my weight until I graduated from college. Looking back, I would say that all of the sports I played in high school helped even more than I realized. I was not as active in school sports in college and began to put on a few extra pounds here and there.

Then I got married, and, as the story goes, a few years later, we were expecting our son. Through my pregnancy, I gained more than just baby weight. I was left with excess weight post-delivery that I was not happy about. This is where my Aunt Cindy really helped me to understand the things that would make a difference. She came to visit us to meet our son shortly after his birth and shared what she was doing with my husband and myself. My husband and I decided to make these changes in our lives too. I was so excited to think this baby weight could start to come off! While my Mom, Sandi, was still in town, she helped us get started in the right direction. By the time our son was two months old, I had lost thirty pounds! I can't begin to tell you how good that felt. Sharing this experience of becoming healthier as new parents and knowing how this would affect for our son's life has been so motivating for us!

## Don Mahrer

I jumped on this journey to better health with my wife, Sandi. I needed to lose a few pounds too. I have to admit this was my first go-around at a healthy lifestyle. I didn't say that this was the first time I needed it. I just said that this was my first time changing my eating habits to gain better health and a thinner me.

When my wife asked me if I would jump on board with her, I knew it was in my best interest to say yes. Little did I know that my life was about to change for the better. When we began, I was thirty pounds overweight. I was also going through a container of Tums every couple of weeks. My wife would write the date on the bottom of the Tums container without me knowing it. She thought I was eating them for candy because the container was empty again so quickly. I had acid reflux so bad that it was difficult for me to lean over at any time. I especially dealt with this during my workday. Just two weeks after we began following the TEID Lifestyle, I was acid reflux free! And yes, I liked the feeling of fitting into my clothes better. This has been a lifestyle change for the better for my wife and me.

# Chapter 12

# STEM CELLS

I want to start out by saying that **we need stem cells**! During the last few years, I have put more attention into researching stem cells and collagen. Our bodies are made up of many different types of cells. Most cells are specialized to perform particular functions, such as red blood cells. They carry oxygen around our bodies in the blood. Stem cells provide new cells for the body as it grows, and replace specialized cells that are damaged or lost. Stem cells can change into other types of cells, according to what the body needs. There are two unique properties that enable them to do this: they can divide over and over again to produce new cells, and as they divide, they can change into the other type of cells that make up the body.

The number of stem cells in younger people is generally much higher than in older people. It has been shown that our production of stem cells decreases after the age of 30, and there is generally a drastic decrease after the age of 60. Stem cell reduction takes place during the aging process, and decreases the body's ability to replenish the tissues and maintain that tissue's (or organ's) original function. Injury and damage can also affect this regardless of age. Therefore, aging is not a matter of the increase in damage, but a matter of failure to replace and repair due to a decreased number of stem cells. Thus, placing those with decreased stem cell production among the greatest known for risk, for most human diseases.

The challenge I was facing was the fact that as we age, our bodies literally slow down the production of stem cells, and if you do still produce them, they are no longer youthful. My skin was suffering from intense sun damage as a teenager, and I was serious about slowing the damage that had been coming to the surface of my skin. I just wasn't sure how to do it. With a focus on a healthy lifestyle, I wanted to reveal it on the outside too.

You have heard or read the talk about collagen. I think finding a great collagen product is one of the greatest dilemmas many of us who are looking have faced. Collagen is a fibrous, supportive protein. It is found in bone cartilage, tendons, ligaments, and skin. It helps skin cells adhere to one another, and also gives the skin strength and elasticity. But here again, the production of collagen also decreases with age, which in turn contributes to skin wrinkling and sagging.

In my study of stem cell injections, which can be quite expensive, I learned that the injected stem cells have a difficult time surviving because of existing inflammation in our bodies. I have experimented personally with stem cell stimulation from whole food products and/or supplements but came to the conclusion that even though this is a benefit to our body nutritionally, it is a slow process.

*It wasn't until a short season ago that my husband (my research buddy) found a product that actually stimulates our bodies to create its own healthy stem cells. I originally deleted this chapter from my book but now that I have answers, I added it back in with the solution!*

What stem cells do:

- Stem cells play a major role in the future of health, wellness, and age reversal.
- They adapt to repair and grow tissue.
- They help your body to create more collagen.
- They help your body reduce inflammation, increase your antioxidants, and build a more youthful and glowing appearance.
- By reducing inflammation, your pain is reduced and balance begins to appear in your body.
- They go to the area of injury or weakness and support your body to heal and strengthen itself.
- They improve sleep, mental clarity, well-being, and overall energy.
- No matter the disease, health issue, or aging symptoms, stimulating your own healthy stem cell production is a win-win!
- And much, much more. Check out the link below to learn more and get your testimony!

Who doesn't want that? Now that I have some answers to our dilemma, I want to share them with everyone I love. Need I say that there is much excitement in our home regarding this product, the health benefits, and the age reversal we are experiencing!

To learn more about re-activating your stem cells go to: **LifeWave.com/JenCin**

# Conclusion:

## Until We Meet Again

I shared deeply and personally with you in this first book because I want you to receive as much of my heart as you could and feel as though we are in this together. My journey may not be your journey, but I pray it gave you a place to begin, as did a variety of the testimonies. I hope you could find yourself inside one of these stories and draw encouragement from someone who has successfully gone before you.

Most importantly, I pray my current lifestyle was inspiring and exciting to you and that you are ready to take on the TEID Lifestyle for yourself. The most important part of this journey for me has been to find you and encourage you to believe in yourself. I want you to discover and know who you are and what you are capable of.

Regardless of what others have said or what you previously felt or thought about yourself, know this one thing, if you have read this far, it tells you that *you are ready for this journey*. Your journal will begin to reveal that you are creating your own testimony of success, just like so many others you read about. And the best part—you are going to take on a whole new confidence about yourself!

In summary, my heart's message to you is quite simple:

- You are loved
- You are worthy of being loved
- This is *your* journey
- Freely and purposefully reach out and take this lifestyle for you
- Open your heart and mind to enjoy every step ahead of you
- Embrace the change with joy
- Know that this is the beginning of your story's new ending
- Believe that your testimony will impact and inspire others
- Love and see yourself for who you truly are
- Know you are beautiful today

**In Conclusion:**

Life is full of ups and downs, failures and accomplishments. There have been tears to cry and laughter to be expressed. If I had missed all of that, it would certainly be an empty life. I am so thankful I get to live my life and not someone else's, which would certainly would not fit me.

I am wonderfully made and have a unique and special purpose. And I am on a journey to uncover it. I am the only one who can fulfill it. I believe everything I need to be who I am called to be is available to me, if not already inside of me.

Sometimes my life makes a lot of sense. Other times I have to go further down the road before hindsight is 20/20. I see it as an adventure. *My adventure.* I do not mind bumps in the road. When I hit a bump I get to take my time going over it and learn from it. I don't have to rush or please others. When ready, I look back to see where I have come from. There are times when I need to rest and process it, but most of the time, I celebrate my journey and who I have become. Sometimes I laugh out loud. Sometimes I laugh at myself. This joy refuels me to keep moving forward. I know that my journey of becoming all I am intended to be will help others. I want them to know that they can be all they are called to be too. I am a vessel of hope, grace, and inspiration. I remember what it has taken me to get here. My heart is so grateful.

**IT IS TIME TO BEGIN YOUR JOURNEY!**

**I CAN'T WAIT TO SEE YOU IN THE NEXT BOOK:**
***"YOU WERE MEANT TO LIVE LIKE THIS"***

# About the Author

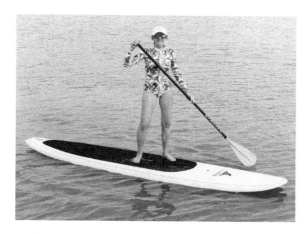

Cindy Brynteson feels her most important titles in life have been wife and mother. She and Jens have been married for forty-six years, and still enjoy being best friends. Living a life of adventure was always the foundation of their home as they raised their two sons. Never would she have imagined the joy they would experience watching these young men grow up, become husbands, and bring two beautiful daughters-in-law into their family. The blessing of becoming "CiCi" to their five incredible grandchildren has been one of her greatest highlights.

Nutrition, fitness, and striving for a healthy balance have always been her passion. It is like she was born for this season of time! As an RN, it was natural to think of ways to support health, healing, and wellness through nutrition and lifestyle. She understands and practices looking for the underlying root issues and supporting the body to repair itself instead of just treating symptoms.

She is and has been a leader in business, ministry, community, and teaching health and wellness. Sharing her success now through the TEID Lifestyle is her honor. Cindy feels she has been given this lifestyle as a gift from God. Her goal is to bring understanding, and simplicity to others that are seeking health, wellness, balance, and weight loss. Her passion and love are contagious and her knowledge runs deep.

For more information, visit **iDietNoMore.com**.

CPSIA information can be obtained
at www.ICGtesting.com
Printed in the USA
BVHW010411151022
649416BV00003B/5